The
Sprouted Peanut Vaccine
and Other Stories

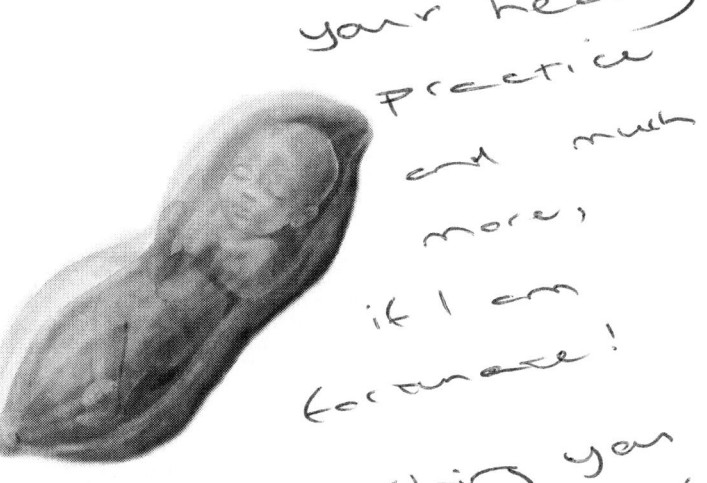

Billy Adam Gottlieb
Illustrated by Seán Newton

Second edition, 2009
First edition, 2008
ISBN 978-0-557-01381-4
Published by lulu.com.

Typeset in Palatino Linotype, Imprint MT Shadow, and Wingdings. Cover and insides © Adam Gottlieb, except "Our Child and Sibling" © Sandra, Richard, and Jonathon Gottlieb, inside illustrations © Seán Newton, created for this book and used with permission, Part Four photos with captions © Price-Pottenger Nutrition Foundation, used with permission, and back cover photo © Rae Allen, used with permission.

The personal stories described herein are true. To protect privacy, names of people other than family members and public figures have been changed, and some details have been omitted.

The information presented is accurate and referenced to the best of the author's ability, and is neither advice nor solicitation. Please consult qualified health professionals before applying any of the content. The author cannot be held responsible for its application or misapplication to another's life.

All rights reserved. No photocopying, scanning, faxing, or other reproducing in whole or in part without signed permission from the author. This protects his ability to earn a living. On the other hand, if you are with a charitable organization that would like a copy but does not have an acquisitions budget, please send your request to:

Billy Adam Gottlieb
book@paplus.net
www.paplus.net

Seán Newton can be reached through www.newtoons.ca.

Contents

Dream	1
Introduction	3

One
Just Peanuts

The Snowball and the Runaway Train	9
Allergy, Anaphylaxis, and Intolerance	10
A Gift	15
Who's a Nut?	19
Peanut Butter to the Rescue!	21
Why Peanuts?	22
Fortress	29
The Frontiers of Science	30
An Experiment	34
The Peanut Detective Squad	35
More Experiments	54
The Full Medical	57
Synthesis	61
The Peanut Detective Bod	63
So What Do You Think?	73
My Game Plan	74

Two
Something Deeper?

Related Symptoms	89
Harmony	92
Related Systems	94
Fire and Water	97
Unexpected Results	98
Unchosen Experiments	100
Hungry Foods	103

Three
From Death to Birth, Life, and Risk
Our Child and Sibling 107
Why Me? 112
The Biology of Stress and Pleasure 123
Going to Seed 125

Four
The Evolutionary Role of Allergy
Turning the Tables 129
Blood Type, Body Type, Feels Good 130
Horny Like the Bull 134
Cancer 135
Wild Speculation 139
Reforming Animal Nature 154

Five
After the Storm, Fertile Calm
Uncrossing Wires 157
The Hypothalamus Who Cried Wolf 159
Some Things Don't Make Sense 161
Sorry I Overreacted 163
Conclusion 164
Feedback 167
Dear Family, Friends, and New Acquaintances 168

Notes 169
Selected Bibliography 201
International and National Allergy Organizations .. 203
Glossary 217
Acknowledgments 225
Index 231

"Let everybody that wants it have it, and make the best use of it."
– *John Harvey Kellogg, on why he didn't patent peanut butter*

Dream

Oh my God, I must have eaten some peanut. Please, please don't let me die. Wait. Hear that? I'm wheezing. See that? I'm red and swollen all over. Am I... am I gonna make it?

(Scream.)

I'm lying in a bed. My bed. It's 4 am. It's been hours since I've eaten. I cooked, from known ingredients. This has happened before.

The Sprouted Peanut Vaccine and Other Stories

Introduction

February 25
"Does it have groundnut in it?"
"It's *fufu*. You'll like it."
"Yeah, I know, but does it have groundnut? It can make me very sick."
"Hold on." (Hollering:) "He doesn't like groundnut!" (Pause.) "The lady says it has a bit."
"Oh, thanks. So I shouldn't have any. Wish I could though. Looks delicious."

March 14
"Would you like some?"
"Sure, as long as there are no peanuts."
"Ohmigod, are you allergic? I'll take it away right now!"
"It's okay. You can keep eating. I just won't have any."
"Yeah, but, like, do you have your medicine?"
"I do – pills and seeds."
"What about Epipen?"
"It doesn't always work that way for me."
"What do you mean…?"

Peanut allergy is a new and sometimes big deal.

I've had many ways of explaining it, and met a wide range of reactions too. It changes from year to year, place to place, and person to person, and in a sense I am fortunate to have had so many experiences. Maybe you've heard about the children who die after eating or breathing a trace of food made or contaminated with peanut, or about the teen killed by the kiss of their beloved who had eaten some.

The lesson I learned, from these and other stories and studies, was to avoid peanuts, carry strong medication, live and travel close to modern hospitals, and wait for a cure. I felt fragile to begin with, in part due to the memory of near-fatal reaction, and this reinforced it. Doubts lingered as to what my body could and couldn't do and what exactly those people had gone through.[1] When I organized my own history, I saw that reaction to a fixed amount of peanut can change with the quality of the ingredient, how it's prepared, with what it's eaten, how I'm feeling, who I'm with, where I am, what time of day it is, whether I know I ate it, and what I do if symptoms appear. This confirmed a hunch that there were other ways of understanding and living this condition, with greater security, even if I couldn't yet articulate them.

I have studied chemistry, environmental toxicology, and traditional Chinese medicine and worked as a lab technician, teacher, journalist, and more.[2] The past two years have been devoted to this inventory of peanut allergy science and making sense of my accidents and experiments, to better move forward and help others do the same.

Peanut allergy can be a complicated, loaded issue. Part One says, let's keep it simple: assume it's only about one food, one disease, and individual people. Part Two picks up the pieces that don't fit and lets them reframe the question. Part Three digests my ancestry and life to date, for clues to the origin and solution of my condition, and raises the question of human ancestry. Part Four fleshes out the last two hundred years of rapid social and environmental change, including the appearance and spread of peanut allergy and related conditions. Part Five summarizes the journey to date and whets an appetite for the future. Together, they explore the terrain between doom and miracle cure:

- ✫ A person can be allergic sometimes but not others;
- ✫ The threshold dose can be as low as one five-thousandth of a peanut, or much higher, and a person can react to the mere thought of peanuts;
- ✫ Reaction can be fatal, debilitating, bothersome, or barely perceptible; anaphylactic, allergic, or intolerant;
- ✫ It can be effectively handled with epinephrine, antihistamine, herbal medicine, meditation, relaxation, emotional support, and/or mere monitoring;

- ☆ Reaction can be made less likely or severe by lifestyle changes including those to nutrition, exercise, environment, and sources of stress and support;
- ☆ Some people outgrow the allergy without doing anything special;
- ☆ Allergy is related to asthma, arthritis, eczema, autism, chronic fatigue, post-traumatic stress, depression, sex addiction, hyperactivity, cancer, and human nature;
- ☆ People may also react to legumes, tree nuts, seeds, cereals, gluten, dairy, eggs, fish, shellfish, pollen, mold, pollution, medicines, perfumes, tampons, fabrics, latex, building materials, pets, insects, energy, and feelings.

Having a reaction can be scary and frustrating. So can having a person empowered to love and help – family, friend, teacher, doctor, or advocate – not believe that they or I can do something about it, as about all illness. For, I need them, and don't want them to have problems either. Of course some problems are natural, and sometimes we just can't change our lives enough to remedy them.

I have tried to use these feelings and experiences to create something good that complements existing books, trade journals, mass media, web sites, and other resources: a thorough analysis of medical and alternative literature, with personal and cultural stories, all written in a clear and fun way, for pre-teens up to seniors; for people who have the allergy or an allergic child, sibling, parent, spouse, lover, schoolmate, coworker, patient, or patron; and from the allergy community to those living with related and unrelated diseases and challenges big and small.

You will find here the tools that have and haven't worked for me, plus many yet to be tried, with an emphasis on using everyday things – like food, drink, activity, rest, elimination, washing, and communicating – as a first resort to jarring, expensive, time-consuming, or hard-to-find products and services. Given allergy as a mismanagement, often under pressure, of routine stimulus, the healing process described herein is a slow and steady destressing and reordering of body and feelings, so as to then be able to handle faster, wilder stuff. All that is needed to begin is to consider that an allergic person's margin of safety may already be, or may be made to be, wider than thought possible, and that facing one's disease is good for it and one's whole quality of life.

As you will find documented here, peanut allergy can be life-threatening, well lived with, improved, outgrown, cured, and/or prevented, in children and adults. It may even be evolution's attempt at solving some even deeper, mightier human health time bomb.

I tried to get this book published through a literary agent and publishing house. Over the course of a year, fifty-some queries and proposals failed. I considered scrapping the project, because of the difficulty ensuring alone that I have accurately interpreted all of the literature and responsibly presented my personal experience; because of the challenge getting this to you and diverse others; and because of the dream of making it big or not all. In the end, I am putting this out on my own account, so that the information and inspiration can be used at least for a while, at least by some. Please take them as possibilities rather than recipes, in a context of support and advice from some key people in your life, including qualified health professionals.

I would be grateful to hear from you as to whether or not this book succeeds and how the content and presentation can be improved. Thank you, and best wishes.

Victoria, Canada
November 2008

One
Just Peanuts

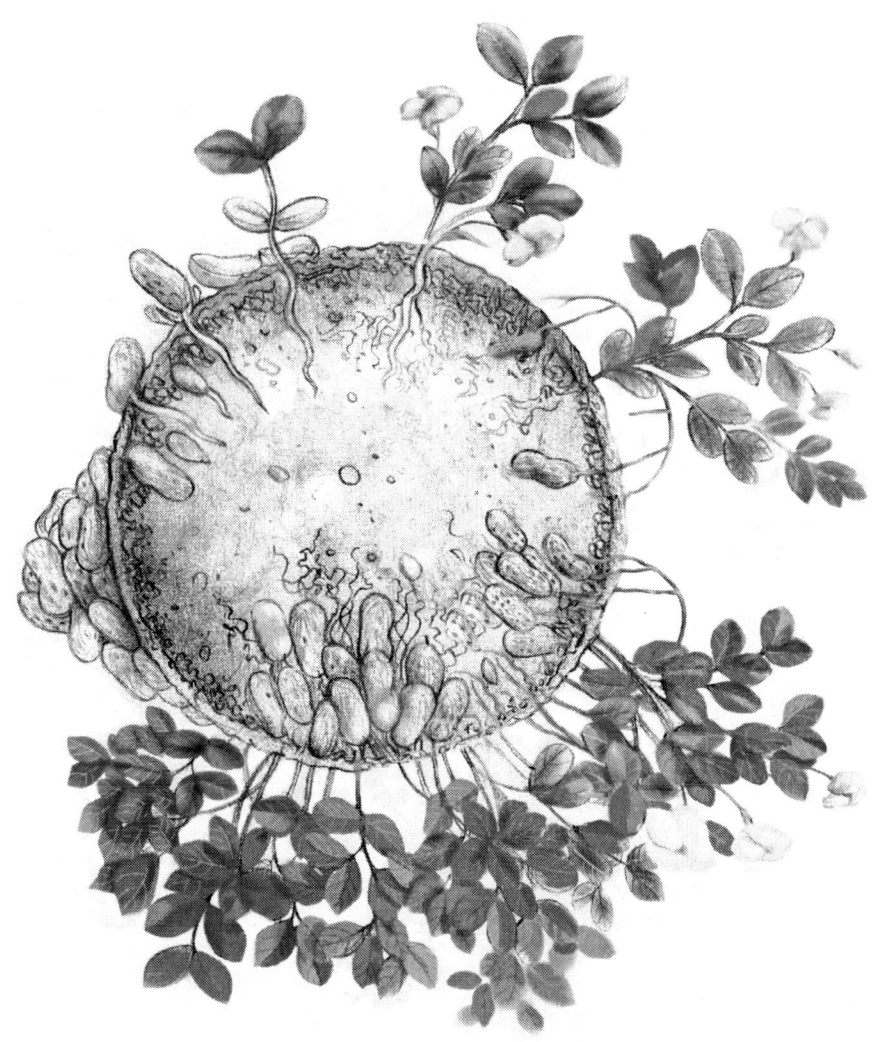

The Sprouted Peanut Vaccine and Other Stories

The Sprouted Peanut Vaccine and Other Stories

The Snowball and the Runaway Train

My lips tingle the second they touch it. Soon comes that sickly irritation at the back of the throat. My eyes puff up, lips swell, and elbow and wrist creases, neck, and back itch, and if I scratch them they break out in glee. I worry I'm losing the battle; my throat tightens, lungs water, and heart races. It feels like a snowball, rolling down a mountain, picking up size and speed until I can't stop it alone. I did or didn't notice the snowflakes that started it.

A child has a rash. Their parent brings them in for an allergy test. It says the child's allergic to peanuts. The tester tells the child to carry an epinephrine injection kit *(Epipen)* at all times, because otherwise they could die at any moment. The parent communicates this to the child's teachers and school directors. The other children learn this way of looking at their classmate and at peanut allergy. The school debates banning peanuts, for the sake of safety and to reduce the risk of being sued. Other nuts are considered suspect too.

If allergy is black-and-white thing – either you don't have it, or you do and any reaction could be fatal – then what is it in onlookers' own bodies and feelings that resonates so strongly with those of someone who is having, has had, or is considered at risk to have an anaphylactic episode?

Allergy, Anaphylaxis, and Intolerance

In surveys across the First World, 1 of every 100 to 200 children and adults reports being allergic to peanuts.[3] It took five years for the number of cases to double in the United States. In Sweden, the level of antibodies associated with immune response to peanut appears to be rising among infants, despite steady levels of peanut consumption.[4]

One in every 4 to 20 Euro-Americans reports some food allergy and/or intolerance in themselves or on behalf of their children. Yet only a fifth to a third of those same people reacts when fed the food under observation.[5] In the United Kingdom, hospital admissions for food allergy increased five-fold in sixteen years, and those for anaphylaxis increased seven-fold. Prescriptions for anaphylaxis increased twelve-fold over roughly the same period. Yet, the population's average level of allergy-specific antibodies did not change.[6] Outside the First World, the situation is less clear.[7]

If the incidence of exposure is not necessarily increasing, then perhaps it is the strength of people's reactions, the rate of reporting, the incidence of emotionally produced *(psychosomatic)* symptoms, the attribution of non-allergy symptoms to allergy, and/or something else.

Whatever the reason, at least a hundred people a year in the US die after eating peanuts or traces thereof.[8] The population as a whole spends four billion dollars on allergy care services and seven billion on prescription drugs – nearly double what they were five years earlier – plus two billion on non-prescription drugs and an unmeasured amount on herbal remedies.[9] Every second citizen takes allergy pills, though not always for allergy symptoms.[10]

There are many definitions of allergy, anaphylaxis, and intolerance. As a scientist, if I had to choose between a peer-reviewed publication and my or someone else's experience of allergy, I should give more credence to the former. So, that's where

I'll start. Out of several texts reviewed, here is one that seems complete and representative:[11]

Intolerance is a "range of reproducible adverse responses to a specific food or food ingredient... This general term includes: allergic reactions; adverse reactions resulting from enzyme deficiencies; pharmacological reactions; and other non-defined responses. Food intolerance does not include food poisoning from bacteria and viruses, moulds, chemicals, toxins, and irritants in foods, nor does it include food aversion. True food intolerance is estimated to affect 5-8% of children... and less than 1-2% of adults. However... as many as 20% of adults believe that they are food intolerant."

Allergy is "an inappropriate reaction by the body's immune system to the ingestion of a food that in the majority of individuals causes no adverse effects. Allergic reactions to foods vary in severity and can be potentially fatal. In food allergy the immune system does not recognize as safe a protein component of the food... This component is termed the allergen. The immune system then typically produces immunoglobulin E *(IgE)* antibodies... which trigger other cells to release substances that cause inflammation. Allergic reactions are usually localised to a particular part of the body and symptoms may include asthma, eczema, flushing, and swelling of tissues or difficulty in breathing. A severe reaction may result in *anaphylaxis*, in which there is a rapid fall of blood pressure and severe shock."[12]

In other words, allergy involves the immune system, and follows an initial, often symptomless, exposure (*sensitization*); intolerance does not necessarily do so. The word "allergy" means "different reactivity" and was first published in 1906, in connection with Clemens von Pircquet's research into a smallpox vaccine; "anaphylaxis" comes from Charles Richet's and Paul Portier's 1902 study of reactions to jellyfish stings, and means "mounting watchfulness."[13] These are distinguished from non-immune reactions, including: *idiosyncratic* ones, like indigestion of milk or fava beans; *pharmacological* ones, like headaches from cheese, red wine, chocolate, or coffee; and *metabolic* ones, like goiter from excessive or poorly processed soy, canola, or cabbage.[14]

In cells as in limbs, inflammation serves to contain a problem, often so that it can be neutralized or expelled before spreading to the rest of the body.[15] The main cells involved in allergic inflammation are *mast cells*, in tissues, and *basophils*, in blood, which technically speaking is also a tissue. The key substances they contain include *histamine, leukotrienes, prostaglandin D_2, and thromboxanes*.[16]

Histamine exists pre-formed in the body. A person's baseline histamine level has to do with their genetics as well as nutrition and lifestyle. Histamine is formed from histidine, an *amino acid* (building block) present in some proteins.[17] It's released into the bloodstream upon exposure to an allergen, then taken up by receptors present in most cells of the body. Uptake can be blocked by H_1-*receptor antagonists*, like diphenhydramine *(Benadryl)*, and H_2-*receptor antagonists*, like ranitidine *(Zantac)*, together known as antihistamines.

On the other hand, leukotrienes, prostaglandin D_2, and thromboxanes are created during allergic reaction. The presence of histamine activates an enzyme that releases stored arachidonic acid, and this in turn is metabolized to leukotrienes, prostaglandin D_2, and thromboxanes. One's baseline level of arachidonic acid has to do with genetics, nutrition, and lifestyle.

Standard medical response to anaphylaxis includes: injecting with adrenaline *(epinephrine)*, to keep blood pressure from dropping and airways from constricting; injecting or orally administering antihistamine, to counter inflammation; giving oxygen; and/or giving fluids intravenously, to improve circulation.[18]

Adrenaline and noradrenaline are things we make naturally to deal with stress: sensors throughout the body inform the hypothalamus gland, in the head; it signals the pituitary, nearby; that sends a messenger to the adrenals; they release the chemicals into blood, to spread rapidly throughout the body.[19]

Allergic reactions have been noted by doctors since at least the mid-1700s. Food allergy has been reported in medical literature since at least the 1920s, though for decades this was sporadic. Experiments on peanut allergy have been done since at least the 1970s.[20]

There is a running debate as to whether or not peanut allergy can simply disappear as a person ages. Some studies find that it cannot, and some writers advise that it cannot, either in principle or to err on the side of caution.[21] Other studies have found that 10% to 25% of people with previous peanut reaction will not react upon voluntarily eating peanut *(oral challenge)*.[22] Some of these people may not truly have resolved, because their previous reactions were unverified self-reports.[23] If a person outgrows peanut allergy, it is likely to be for good, especially if their reactions were mild in the first place and if they keep in practice eating peanuts.[24]

Less has been written about what someone can do to initiate the process. Successful immunotherapy has been documented since at least the 1930s.[25] It often involves getting a person used to tiny doses of the allergen and then working them up to amounts they are likely to encounter in foods. It may be combined with diet, as with massage, fasciatherapy, muscle testing, acupuncture, chiropractic, and other treatments to resolve deep-set physical-emotional tension.[26] As we speak, Chinese herbs, IgE-scavenging injections, and other cures are also being tried.[27] There's even research to harness accidental remedies, like that of a boy who stopped being allergic to peanuts after receiving a bone marrow transplant intended to boost his immune system.[28]

In terms of preventing newborns and others from becoming allergic in the first place, vaccines are being developed, for example using mutated peanut proteins. Meanwhile, nutrition and lifestyle continue to be debated – particularly, as to whether or not pregnant and nursing mothers need to avoid eating peanuts. More about this in a couple of chapters.

For all of these people, experiments are being done to develop allergy-free *(hypoallergenic)* peanuts.[29]

The likelihood that someone is or will be allergic to peanuts can be tested in various ways. A common test involves putting a drop of peanut extract on the forearm, pricking the skin, and seeing if hives appear. Extract is used because there is a small risk of systemic reaction to pure peanut. This skin-prick test can have *false positives*: people who have outgrown allergy, or been exposed to an allergen but never had whole-body symptoms, may test positive. Perhaps 90% of people who test positive aren't actually allergic. Including salt water as a negative control and histamine as a positive control can help give correctly interpretable results. Another test is the *radioallergosorbent (RAST)* one. It searches for peanut-specific IgE in blood. It is less sensitive and not necessarily more accurate than the skin-prick test, and can have *false negatives*. These are more dangerous than false positives: perhaps 20% of people who are actually allergic to peanut would not seem to be from their RAST result. The modified *CAP RAST* may be more accurate. The only truly systemic test, and the one that gives the most reliable results, is a *placebo-controlled* oral challenge: eating a food known to possibly contain peanut, under medical supervision. It is considered risky for people with a history of anaphylaxis; for this reason, and perhaps given the liability it implies, it is not as common as some of the other tests.[30]

A Gift

I have always felt a need to help the world suffer less. Looking back at the world in which I grew up, and at how my body was then, I feel unnamed stresses and hear much talk about the state of the world, who is to blame, and what must be done. We are activists who often fight amongst ourselves and bystand collective movements, speaking rarely of injustices done to us or of our value to the world.

In my college years, aboriginal people's movements in Canada make some historic, public gains. When I get out, I'm drawn to them. The way I see it at first, I'm among the most privileged class of people here and they're among the least, so I have something to offer them. I don't know much about my own ethnic group, and don't want to know. Soon enough, though, their wars, epidemics, dispossession, assimilation, and fallout of depression and self-abuse teach me about our Holocaust and exile, and stir up some mighty feelings I didn't even know I had.

I start visiting my own elders and archives, and found an aboriginal-solidarity program on community radio. It's both a burden and a relief to my burdens. It gives me the chance to interview people from all over the world, whose lives are so different from mine, yet with whom I get along with surprising ease. I say "surprising" because I've had an image of being abnormal or wrong, and of this peanut allergy is an epitome: "why does he make such fusses, and how come he gets special treatment?" If I wasn't that different to begin with – just manifesting something scary that anyone may be capable of – the labels widen the gap, and food reactions are key moments in learning to feel alone.

One day, a colleague suggests I invite this guy Harvey to the show. She doesn't say much more about him. We arrange a meeting. Odd fellow, I think. Never met anyone like him. Not too sure about putting him on-air. Go for it.

The show is his testimony about living with HIV/AIDS and teaching aboriginal people how to prevent and cope with it.[31] At one point, he says something that I just can't get my head around: he feels the illness is a gift he's received. He contracted it from unsafe sex or drug injection, and took it as a wake-up call to stop that self-abuse. It took a "death sentence" to give his life a purpose: to be lived, and help others live.

Meanwhile I've mostly wanted to be rid of peanut allergy, and indeed all illness; to see myself as healthy, be treated as normal, and share food without restriction. Curiously, none of my family or friends has ever expressed a strong desire for me to be rid of it. They may try to protect me, but not rescue me, from it. Peanut sensitivity, it seems, is part of the person they love. Especially given my at-times fierce independence, it is a vulnerability that lets them into my life. And it may enlighten them as much as anything I can consciously teach. This allergy reminds me who I am and for whom I'm responsible. Like an old friend, it may visit from time to time, and some of those times I can cut short or put off the visit. Sometimes I shoo my friend away because I want to be alone and no longer fear feeling it; sometimes I choose other company.

If I don't like how someone responds to my allergy, maybe I'll assert absolute authority: "you don't know, only I know, and you have to let me do what I want because otherwise I'll get sick." I've heard similar things from people with allergies and other mysteriously disabling conditions, like fibromyalgia. And I've heard them from our caregivers, sometimes even more radically. Maybe that's what it takes to get these conditions taken seriously. But something bugs me about it: like someone's making my case out to be more hopeless and scary than it is, to make theirs seem more manageable. I sometimes do that to other people and use my "strengths" to feel better about my "weaknesses."

In the moment of reaction, in my identity as an "allergic" person, and otherwise, I have often felt invaded. It hurts twice as bad coming from a loved one or authority. I've had trouble distinguishing their ideas and sensations from mine, and, when pressed, have sometimes misrepresented what is going on in my body, to tell the story they seem to want to hear. Allergy and depression have felt like one part of me fighting with another – as if nutrients were bound to poisons, or someone else's past to my present. There are obvious crises but these come from an underlying condition.

September 19

I've been extra active lately, yet eating light. On the way to the pool tonight this old voice goes off in my head: "you can't go on like this! What are you trying to do? You gotta eat more protein. And you need carbs to get energy!" I've been practicing waiting out the fuss, to feel what I want here and now. Tonight I want to swim. So I do, for even longer than usual, and then make a simple supper. I feel good. But it's amazing how much sway those voices can have.

What I'm irritated by peanuts or something else, what I want to hear is, "this is not just about you. I may have felt something similar before. Here's how I feel trying to care for you…" In general, I haven't often heard "no" or felt the license to say it. It's been a struggle to learn appropriate social boundaries, and this has been vital to my self-worth. It's been a relief to meet people who can name and share the challenges of finding one's place in a rapidly changing society – like growing up with parents and grandparents away most of the time and/or reacting against previous generations seen as too authoritarian.

October 7

I feel invaded by Anna and don't tell her. Suddenly it's too much and I shut her out: turn cold, move away, refuse food. My gut tightens. Where have I felt that before? With Mom, long ago. She keeps bringing up how I'd push her away when seemingly needing comfort. "Not like other kids." Why does it have to be me who's the problem? Maybe she needed something too. I didn't want to hurt her, but couldn't let her in. If I didn't speak up or act out, in the heat of the moment, I could at least set an internal boundary and retreat into my world. One of my brothers says I had some borderline autistic behaviours. But the feelings would have to go somewhere.

Who's a Nut?

Peanuts are seeds of a plant in the legume family, alongside lentils, chickpeas, soy, dry beans, string beans, alfalfa, clover, lupines, tamarind, carob, vetch, and more. According to the *Linnaeus* botanical system, they're a family because they look and act similarly, as confirmed later by genetic testing.

Most of the legume food plants are of Indo-Middle Eastern or northwest South American origin, domesticated some 2500 to 5000 years ago.[32] Many are small, reproduce by seedpods, have cleft leaves in groups of three, and, in their roots, host bacteria which have the special ability to take inorganic nitrogen from the air and turn *(fix)* it into organic nitrogen. Plants and animals need organic nitrogen to build the proteins that balance carbohydrates. A balance of nitrogen and carbon is also needed for proper decay *(composting)* of plant and animal matter into soil, to complete the cycle of life's renewal.

Peanut plants have the curious feature of flowers that turn to *pegs* that, in turn, dig into the ground, where seedpods emerge.[33] Hence the nickname, *groundnut*. Peanuts aren't related to the Bambara groundnut that is native to Africa, and aren't nuts in the sense of seeds or pits of tree-borne fruit like walnut, almond, or cashew.[34]

The seed is 40 to 55 percent fat (oil), 20 to 55 percent protein, and 10 to 20 percent carbohydrate, depending on the variety and growing conditions. It also has *tannins* (bitter compounds also found in tea, wine, and some fruit), vitamins such as B_3, B_9, and E, and minerals such as boron, calcium, copper, iron, magnesium, manganese, molybdenum, phosphorus, potassium, and zinc, and tends to accumulate toxic minerals like cadmium and lead.[35]

From the New World, peanuts spread to Europe and Africa, by the early 1500s, and to Southeast Asia, by the early 1600s.[36] Today, they are a staple crop for millions of people in tropical, subtropical, and semi-arid climates, and the fourth most important oilseed worldwide.[37] They are mostly used as food and livestock feed, and to make food oil and cosmetics. India, China, the United States,

Nigeria, and Senegal produce three-quarters of the planet's peanuts.[38] Indonesian *satay*, Thai *phad thai*, Chinese *kung pao*, Senegalese *maffé*, Brazilian *vatapá*, Mexican *mole*, and American chili are some of the dishes often or always flavoured, thickened, and/or fortified with peanuts. Brittle, cookies, sundaes, and chocolates are some of the sweets. Peanut oil is prized for salads and deep frying. And peanuts find their way, deliberately or accidentally, into a host of other homemade, restaurant, and packaged foods.

It's hard to know exactly when and how peanuts started being eaten by people in what is now the First World, where most allergy is reported. Spanish and Portuguese settlers noted indigenous people eating them raw, roasted, or smoked and using them for oil or medicine. Early African-Americans had them raw, roasted, and boiled, among other ways; Euro-Americans ate them too but often reported intolerance and considered the food undignified.[39] Peanuts became an important US crop in the early 1800s; mechanized farming and processing became possible in the late 1800s and early 1900s; these and other market and government factors led to a consumption boom. Peanuts are now one of the country's top ten crops, and are eaten by most of its citizens.[40] Their popularity in the United Kingdom is more recent, dating from the mid 1900s, after the Second World War.[41] In the latter 1900s and early 2000s, the way peanuts are bred, grown, and/or consumed has continued to evolve.

Peanut Butter to the Rescue!

Peanut butter was supposed to be made for people like me.

In the latter 1800s, Seventh Day Adventists tried to reform an America rife with malnutrition, libidinousness, and other ills, using Sylvester Graham's crackers, William Keith Kellogg's cereal flakes, and his brother John Harvey's "prepared nut meal." Each was meant to balance the energetic highs and lows of refined carbs and help their worst victims, from tuberculosis patients to elders who had lost their teeth to decay.

It was hard work spreading the word of mouth and grinding the nuts by hand, but, by and by, Joseph Lambert and Ambrose Straub patented peanut butter machines, Joseph "Skippy" Rosefield made them churn smoother, and Rosefield introduced partially hydrogenated oil, to keep the product from separating and spoiling on the shelf. Other folks mechanized peanut sowing, weeding, harvesting, sorting, shelling, blanching, and roasting. George Washington Carver and company showed that growing peanuts in rotation with cotton could save that crop from pests and replenish soil, and that the nuts could be used for anything from paper to ink, glue, lubricants, and plastics. Farming was subsidized, imports were restricted, prices dropped, bread-slicing machines appeared, mass media and marketing blossomed, and the peanut butter sandwich, "cup," and chocolate bar were born. During the Second World War, when many domestic high-energy foods were rationed and foreign ones were unavailable, peanuts flowed freely and were fed to the army. Today, peanut butter is found in 85% of US homes, and Americans eat a hundred times more of the stuff per person than they did a century ago.[42]

Actually, the Incas of what is now northwest South America were peanut butter fans centuries ago, and their ancestors may have been the first to domesticate the plant. Unfortunately, we don't have any record of their patents or *per-capita* consumption.

Why Peanuts?

Peanut allergy is a potentially spectacular illness, and there is a lively debate as to how it works and how, therefore, to stop it. Some researchers and advocates focus on a single cause, while others consider many co-factors.[43] Most focus on allergic substances; some also emphasize genetics and lifestyle; and a few include feelings and energy.[44]

This chapter presents twenty-seven theories culled from over a hundred sources. It gives references only for some of the obscurer notions, which may beg fuller explanation. Factual assessment of the theories, with all the references, is left to a later chapter. In this way, you have time to ponder which theories make the most and least sense, how they fit together, and what ground all fail to cover.

Something natural about peanuts

Allergies are due to **proteins**. In the case of peanuts, the main ones include vicilin *(Ara h 1)*, conglutin *(Ara h 2)*, and glycinin *(Ara h 3, Ara h 4)*.[45] For this reason, as discussed earlier, genetic modification of peanut protein is part of the research toward vaccines and hypoallergenic seed varieties (*cultivars*).

There may also be allergens in peanut **oil**.

Specifically, peanuts are rich in **arachidonic acid**, a fatty acid whose metabolites include inflammatory agents of allergy: leukotrienes, prostaglandin D_2, and thromboxanes.[46] Chronic overconsumption of arachidonic acid congests and inflames a person's body in a way that predisposes them to allergy and possibly related, degenerative diseases like arthritis and cancer.[47]

Food allergies are due to aromatic compounds known as **phenols** (or *phenolics*). The suspect ones in peanuts are phenyl isothiocyanate, piperine, and vanillylamine.[48]

One subgroup of phenols, ***salicylates***, is responsible for allergies to peanuts and some other foods.[49]

Peanuts can develop allergenic (and carcinogenic) molds, ***aflatoxins***, during growth, storage, and processing.[50] These have been termed the US peanut industry's number one problem, leading to changes in how peanuts are bred and grown.[51]

There is something that peanuts have in common with all **legumes** that makes them allergens.

Peanuts have some allergen in common with all **nuts**.

Foods which come from the reproductive parts of plants contain higher concentrations of allergenic **pollens**. This includes the seedpod legumes (like peanuts and beans), seed cereals (like wheat and corn), pit or seed fruit, seed vegetables, flower vegetables (like artichoke and broccoli), and tubers, as opposed to leaf and stem vegetables (like lettuce and celery). It extends to the products of animals that eat these parts of plants (like honey, or grain-fed fish, meat, dairy, and eggs).

Pollens from one kind of plant can make people allergic to related or unrelated plant and animal foods. An example of such *concomitance* is more reported legume and cereal allergy during grass pollination season.[52]

Peanuts are one of the harder legumes to digest. Moreover, people with certain **genetic natures** have an extra hard time digesting them. This may have to do with their ethnicity, and can be recognized by certain physical and emotional traits. In traditional East Indian *(Ayurvedic)* medicine, for example, people who are relatively *pitta* (fiery, as typified by a muscular build or loud presence) or *vata* (airy, often thin and nervous) are discouraged from eating peanuts, which may exaggerate their natures to the point of illness, whereas peanuts healthily balance out *kapha* (watery, often corpulent and grounded) folks.[53]

Something about how peanuts are grown

Peanuts are often grown in rotation with corn and **cotton**.[54] The latter can be treated with **pesticides** not approved for food plants, whether because they are too toxic or their food safety has not been verified. Much of the chemical goes into the soil and then into the plants next grown there. Most pesticides are soluble in oil rather than water, so they concentrate *(bioaccumulate)* in the fatty tissues of plants, like nuts and seeds. They further concentrate and provoke diseases in the fatty tissues (like breasts and liver) of animals that eat them. They also wind up in the liver because that is a key organ of detoxification, and the body recognizes pesticides as foreign substances. In its effort to metabolize them, for example to make them easier to excrete, the liver can turn the chemicals into other substances *(metabolites)* that have their own toxicity.

Peanuts have some of the highest **pesticide residues** of any food.⁵⁵ The residues may be explained in several ways. For one, peanuts are a relatively fatty food, so they uptake a lot of pesticide. For another, peanuts are a commercially important crop. If it fails, money is lost; to prevent disease, high doses and/or extra potent chemicals are used, and a genetically narrow range of hardy, productive cultivars is developed; over time the target pests learn to become resistant; spraying and breeding are intensified; and the spiral continues.

Intensive, selective breeding of peanuts and other food plants, whether by traditional or novel methods, may give them harmful properties.⁵⁶

Something about how peanuts are consumed

Many cultures, for example in West Africa and Southeast Asia, have a long history of eating peanuts, with no reported allergy. If allergy rates are rising among First-World Caucasians, it is because they are consuming peanuts in **quantities and forms** that are **unprecedented** for them, for the original inhabitants of those climates, or even for longtime peanut-eating cultures.⁵⁷ An example is pre-manufactured, dry roasted peanut butter with additives, as opposed to fresh or boiled whole peanuts.⁵⁸

Once someone is sensitized to peanuts, **repeated exposure** will worsen *(potentiate)* their reaction.

If a woman consumes **peanuts while pregnant**, her child is more likely to develop a peanut allergy.

If an **infant** is **introduced** to peanuts **too young**, they can have an allergic reaction then or be more likely to develop one later. This is because it takes time for them to develop the ability to digest various foods, and for their immune systems to discern toxins from nutrients.[59]

Something about lifestyle

Nowadays, our immune systems are bombarded with untraditional forms of **radiation**, from power lines, appliances, and so on. This can impede their development and functioning, and allergy is one result. Exposure in the womb may be particularly risky.[60]

Much the same goes for certain **vaccines**, or for excessive vaccination as a whole. Many vaccines are disease-causing microorganisms (like bacteria and viruses) in a modified, weakened, or killed form: not enough to cause disease, but enough for the immune system to learn to oppose. The allergy problem may come from exposing people to illnesses in unusual form, by unusual route (like bloodstream injection instead of food, water, or air), or by unusual progression (suddenly, at a certain age, instead of progressively, from birth). It may also have to do with side ingredients in the vaccines.

An early **bout of** bacterial or viral **illness**, like chicken pox or strep throat, can also disturb immune system development.[61]

So can **nurturing** an infant **with formula or cow's milk**, whether in place of or in addition to breastfeeding. There may also be a problem with preserving breast milk for later drinking.

Our **air, water, and food** are more **polluted** now than ever before. This includes physical pollutants (like dust) and chemical ones (like heavy metals). Pollution taxes immune, detoxification, and other systems to the point of causing or worsening allergy and other illnesses. Air pollution in particular may provoke asthma and make related conditions, like allergy, more common. This includes contamination of outdoor air (by things like factory and car emissions) and indoor air (by volatile synthetics in furniture, paint, and other materials), as compounded by "sick building:" the creation of closed environments in which pollutants are recycled, oxygen depletes, carbon dioxide accumulates, mold grows, and so on.[62]

At the same time, in the First World especially, many foods and living **environments** are more **sanitized** than they used to be. A certain amount of dirt, microbes, and other challenges to our immune and detox systems is necessary for their development and ongoing fitness. If those systems are left idle, they may overreact to legitimate threats or invent threats, like normally innocuous foods, to keep themselves busy.[63]

A precondition to the development of allergy is **clogging of the liver**. The liver gets clogged by intense, abundant food, drugs, pollution, stress, work, and even emotions sustained in one's lifetime or by one's recent ancestors. It's unclogged by appropriate nutrition, fasting, fitness, rest, calm, and so on. Modern living has upset the traditional balance between the two, in favour of clogging. Over the long term, this impairs vital functions of the liver and its partner, the gallbladder, like separating nutrients from toxins and producing the bile to digest fat.[64] It also taxes the kidneys and adrenal glands, which among other things are needed to handle stress, detoxify the blood, and – according to traditional

Chinese medicine – reenergize the liver. So liver health spirals down.

Sluggish digestion and overeating, in general, can give someone a "**leaky gut:**" the intestines are full of partly decomposed food; some seeps back into the body; allergens that normally get eliminated harmlessly go places they shouldn't (like the *interstitial* fluid which surrounds cells and allows them to exchange substances with blood); and the immune system identifies the allergens as invaders and tries to deal with them, but in a way that may make things worse. This explains symptoms like lymph node swelling and itching.[65]

A person can be so **afraid** of an allergy or other illness, whether or not they have had it before, that they can develop its symptoms without being exposed.

Fortress

Dream. I've been living in Zambia, for long enough now, in the same place and with the same people, to feel comfortable. We're a small group of foreigners and locals, living in a kind of retreat centre, modestly but still differently from the villagers. For the first time in a while, I leave the compound, with teammates, to go to the city. I've been restless to go off on my own of late. Will I make a break for it now? Out in the big world, I start to remember how it feels to be this vulnerable – and the times I bolted, thrilled, and then panicked.

When I landed in Africa, it was like the mistrust I had always carried back home got turned up a notch so I could hear it. I packed medicines, wore hard-to-pickpocket pants, kept moving, dressed not-rich, and toughened my talk (while also being basically kind and open). I had grown up in fear of going out into the world, what with peanut allergy and a family vibe of being marginal. I'd wanted to fit in but chosen to live in ways that made it harder, then even consoled myself by celebrating the difference thus exaggerated. Over time I built and armed a fortress, to defend clan and self. I often acted like I didn't need anyone; then, finding myself and us alone and not under threat, counted my possessions – coins, hockey cards, candy, whatever – and imagined they were worth more than they were, so I could less afford to share them. At the same time, I exposed and rubbed salt in my wounds: got pierced, skipped meals when hungry, gave away gifts received, and so on. I despaired of ever feeling full and connected, and blew hot and cold like they say my granddaddy did.

I've been on a mission to feel healthy, all the while fearing I may never get there. "Healthy enough" means able and deserving to make it in the world.

The Frontiers of Science

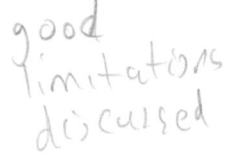
good limitations discussed

It is not easy to get a good toxicologist to support a claim you may have that some substance causes a certain disease. For better or for worse, conservatism is built into the scientific method in many ways.

The suspected cause has to be checked out by deliberate experiment, involving one *(case)* group of people who are exposed to it and a similar *(control)* group who are not.

For ethical reasons, all participants *(subjects)* must be consenting. For legal reasons this usually means they're adults.

In order to claim that the results apply to all people, a large number of subjects is needed, and they must have a wide range of ages, ethnicities, occupations, and/or other demographics, depending on what's being studied.

Subjects have to be assigned at random to the case and control groups, to make sure that any outside factors *(confounding variables)* apply equally to both. Both subject and experimenter must be unaware *(double-blind)* as to who is getting what treatment. This is to prevent them from biasing results by finding what they expect *(placebo effect)*.

The exposure *(dose)* level and timing pattern must be close to what an ordinary person would experience in real life. Yet the subjects shouldn't be harmed, and the experiment can't last so long that participants drop out (which would reduce statistical validity) or change too much physically (which would introduce confounding variables).

Results *(responses)* must be objectively measurable, in numbers *(quantitatively)* rather than in descriptions *(qualitatively)*, and analyzed by statistical tests agreed on by scientists.

These tests can prove only whether or not a certain dose is associated *(correlates)* with a certain response, not if one causes the other.

The Sprouted Peanut Vaccine and Other Stories

Successful correlations may be considered for publication in a peer-reviewed journal. For the scientific community to accept them as fact, they must be reproduced by many independent researchers.

Failed correlations may not be considered results, in the sense of disproving the theory *(hypothesis)* with which the experiment started out.

The answer to uncertainty is often "more research," even when the uncertainty has more to do with funding or politics than with science.

If we wanted to study peanut allergy, and considered that only such science were valid, we could probably go no further, for the following additional reasons.

Live, human subjects are generally forbidden. Exceptions include a consenting volunteer receiving treatment for a terminal illness, or a person paid to try an as-yet unlicensed drug. However, even this may imply some coercion, for example financial need, thus neither true consent nor randomness. And how to learn about children, who are the main victims of peanut allergy?

It is expensive, time-consuming, and logistically challenging to study a big and diverse group of people. Only certain kinds of researchers may have such means, and this may introduce biases. For example, a well-known and -funded institution might be cautious about taking on or publishing work that is controversial or leads to results not immediately clear.

Only once results are obtained can they be acted upon, such as by making a remedy available to the public.

Real-life doses that cause problems are often small or moderate and long-term *(chronic,* as in home or workplace air, water, or food), as opposed to high and unique *(acute,* as by accident). These can be hard to reproduce experimentally, due to funding, confounding variables, and other issues.

Many behaviours are hard to measure with numbers. Forcing a poor-fitting, numerical lens upon them may distort how results are interpreted and discard qualitative results of great value.

Many people want to know the cause, not just the correlation, so that they can take action: make lifestyle changes, file a workers' compensation or class-action lawsuit, and so on.

Publication in a peer-reviewed journal adds more time to the process and may add bias, in the sense that a given journal may favour certain kinds of studies, writing, or author credentials. Most journals are not circulated to the general public or written in language that's easy to understand.

For many topics, like peanut allergy, there is so much literature that even the most experienced specialist may not know it all and so be able to tell readers and patients the full range of ideas out there, or which are most likely true.

It is hard to reproduce results which do not get published, are inaccurately reported or interpreted, or whose experimental method is not fully disclosed, for example because of a pending patent.

We could, as is commonly done, study small animals, like mice, to which humans are distantly related. But then we'd have to prove that the results apply to us. Many diseases do not cross species lines. The psychosomatic factor, in particular, may work very differently, and be hard to understand, in non-humans.

We could also study people after they have been exposed *(epidemiologically)* by accident. At least then we'd have realistic subjects and doses, so perhaps more license to generalize. However, we couldn't control many confounding variables, so it would be hard to confirm or deny almost any explanation of the results. This alone can stifle otherwise compelling evidence. Consider the dozens of years and thousands of deaths it took for scientists, governments, and companies to accept and act upon the facts that smoking causes lung cancer and seatbelts save lives.

If a phenomenon has to be so obvious and to have done so much damage in order to pass the hurdles of institutional science, what are the odds of understanding and healing something as freaky as peanut allergy? And what is the public value of such science, especially when it is funded with taxpayers' money?

The situation seems ripe for extreme responses – like quick-fix medicines or lawsuits – that may only further obscure and delay simple, effective learning and action, using tools already known.

Still, I want science to be part of the solution. And I can do what any scientist who wants to get well and help others may do: volunteer to be one ethical, realistic, subjective, statistically insignificant subject.

An Experiment

Last Fall a friend gave me some organic seed peanuts for the garden. Now it's Spring and I'm looking at the bag wondering… if these aren't exactly the sort of high-quality peanuts I want to try eating!

I shell a couple and, over the next few days, sprout them. The sprouts smell good, alive and fresh like other legume and non-legume sprouts I've had and unlike the peanut smell I have usually associated with danger. I eat a piece of one. It tastes fine too! I breathe normally, with a mild hard feeling in my gut.

The Peanut Detective Squad

Back to solving the peanut allergy problem, rationally.

Given few case-control studies on whole people, what can I do? Build a case on each theory, using biological principles, case-control studies on human cells and whole animals, and stories *(anecdotes)* of people's experiences, using a framework such as:

- ☆ The charge: does the theory refer to an anaphylactoid/allergenic substance, or rather to a precondition to the development of anaphylaxis/allergy?
- ☆ Direct evidence: has it been found to produce the range of symptoms typical of peanut anaphylaxis/allergy?
- ☆ Corroborating evidence: has it been found on the scene of anaphylaxis/allergy to other substances, and away from safe substances?
- ☆ Motive: is there a biological explanation?
- ☆ Exculpatory evidence: are there important confounding variables?

Consider substances commonly associated with allergy. The main ones are peanuts, tree nuts, fish, and shellfish. A fuller list includes:[66]

- ☆ Foods: banana, cod, corn, cottonseed, cow's milk, egg (white and yolk), guava, mandarin, okra, pea, peach, peanut, rice, sesame, shrimp, soy, strawberry, tomato, wheat;
- ☆ Food additives: sulfites;
- ☆ Stings and bites: bee, fire ant, jellyfish, snake, wasp;
- ☆ Other plant, animal, and fungal matter: pollen, dander, mold;
- ☆ Medicines: aspirin, penicillin-type antibiotics, some surgical anaesthetics or relaxants;
- ☆ Other chemicals: latex.

For reasons already discussed, use only studies that are peer reviewed and apparently free of profit motive (for example, by government, academic, or public health agencies rather than advocacy groups, private practitioners, or health product sellers). To find them, use Bowker's directory of books in print, periodical databases like Medline and PsychInfo, and the Google internet search engine.

Now I have read the major books on peanut allergy and most of the articles to which they refer, as well as many others. In the endnotes to this chapter, you'll find over a hundred references. The goal is to get an idea of what's out there and how to make sense of it. Always, there will be other studies, interpretations, and ways of organizing the information.

Something natural about peanuts

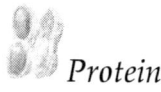 *Protein*

Charge: Substance.

Direct evidence: Yes. People and laboratory animals dosed with peanut protein can have allergic reactions.[67] When peanut protein is partly or completely broken down *(hydrolyzed)* into its amino acids, allergy may be milder or absent entirely.[68]

Corroborating evidence: Maybe. Allergenic legumes, nuts, and animal products tend to resemble peanuts in the proportion, though not necessarily the sequence, of the various amino acids.[69] Some non-allergens do too. Some of the allergenic legumes and nuts contain vicilin, conglutin, and/or glycinin, specifically.[70]

Motive: Yes. Isolated human cells exposed to peanut protein produce IgE.[71] This may require other factors *(co-factors)* to be present. Peanut protein is rich in the amino acids phenylalanine (used by the body to make adrenaline) and histidine (a precursor to histamine), both important allergy biochemicals.[72]

Exculpatory evidence: Yes. The allergic effect of peanut protein is affected by heat processing, as occurs in dry roasting and curing.[73] The foods with common amino acid profiles can share other suspect properties, like aflatoxin.

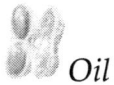 *Oil*

Charge: Substance.

Direct evidence: Yes. There are many reports of allergy to peanut oil in food and cosmetics.[74]

Corroborating evidence: Maybe. Peanut oil is roughly one-fifth saturated, three-fifths monounsaturated, and one-fifth polyunsaturated.[75] Specifically, it is high 16-carbon saturates, 18-carbon monounsaturates, and 18-carbon diunsaturates.[76] Pure oils that share this profile – like *oleic* canola, used in food, and almond, used in cosmetics – are not commonly reported allergens.[77] However many whole foods that share it, are: tree nuts (whose proportion and amount of the various fats tends to resemble peanuts'); legumes (which have similar proportions but much lower amounts); and animal products, like dairy, eggs, and fish (which have somewhat similar proportions and amounts).

Motive: Maybe. I have not found an explanation of how these fatty acids can provoke anaphylaxis or allergy in the moment, as opposed to contributing to general inflammation of the body.

Exculpatory evidence. Yes. Crude, cold-pressed, and non-food-grade peanut oils tend to contain protein and other impurities.[78] Peanut oil that has been refined with heat and solvents tends not to, and to be safe for people-allergic people.[79]

 Arachidonic acid

Charge: Substance.

Direct evidence: Maybe. I have not found a study of anaphylaxis/allergy in people or animals dosed with pure arachidonic acid.

Corroborating evidence: Yes. Most of the foods rich in arachidonic acid – muscle meat, dairy, eggs, shellfish, peanuts, and nori seaweed, but not other legumes, other seaweeds, and nuts – are associated with allergy.[80] Peanut-allergic people may react more often or more intensely to animal products than do people without peanut allergy.[81] Some low arachidonic acid foods, such as wheat and soy, are commonly reported allergens, while others are not.

Motive: Yes. Arachidonic acid is used by the body to make prostaglandin D$_2$, leukotrienes, and thromboxanes, which are key agents of allergic inflammation.

Exculpatory evidence: Yes. The high arachidonic acid foods can share other suspect properties, like protein.

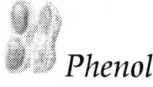 *Phenol*

Charge: Substance.

Direct evidence: Maybe. People who are allergic to a food can react adversely to its pure phenols, and be healed by immunotherapy using them.[82] I haven't found a study of how non-allergic people respond to those phenols.

Corroborating evidence: Maybe. Among foods having at least two of the three phenols suspected in peanut allergy, some are common allergens (cow's dairy, egg, legumes) and some are not (banana, chocolate, grapes, meats, nightshades, nutmeg, onions).[83] Many common allergens, such as wheat and corn, do not have any of the three, but have others.

Motive: Yes. Phenols lengthen the time adrenaline stays in circulation and intensify its stimulation of the heart and intestines, to the point of producing intestinal contractions *(peristalsis)* and racing heart *(tachycardia)*, both symptoms of anaphylaxis.[84]

Exculpatory evidence: No. The phenols tested are single compounds, free of impurities.

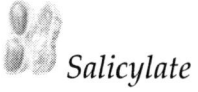 *Salicylate*

Charge: Substance.

Direct evidence: Yes. Hives, eczema, asthma, and anaphylaxis to salicylates in food and aspirin have been reported.[85]

Corroborating evidence: Maybe. Salicylates are common in fruits, vegetables, nuts, and spices; a few of these are common allergens but most are not.[86]

Motive: Maybe. Salicylate sensitivity is often considered an intolerance, not an allergy, as it does not involve IgE. It may involve histamine.[87]

Exculpatory evidence: Yes. These foods can contain other suspect properties, like aflatoxin.

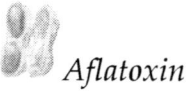 *Aflatoxin*

Charge: Substance.

Direct evidence: Yes. Aflatoxin can trigger asthma, weaken the immune system, cause developmental *(teratogenic)* defects in children and farm animals, and cause cancer to the liver, lungs, and other organs.[88] Aflatoxin in peanut meal, specifically, can kill farm animals.[89]

Corroborating evidence: Yes. Cigarette smoke and mold, which contain aflatoxin, can produce anaphylaxis and asthma and potentiate allergy.[90] Most of the foods prone to aflatoxin (like legumes, cereals, tree nuts, black pepper, and milk) are common allergens; the few that are not (like ginger and cloves) tend to be eaten in much smaller amounts.[91]

Motive: Yes. Aflatoxin can produce an IgE response and damage the main organs and systems involved in allergy.[92]

Exculpatory evidence: Yes. The way a crop is grown, processed, and stored may affect other properties. For example, prolonged storage of foods rich in polyunsaturated oils can yield carcinogenic free radicals.[93] The toxicity of cigarette smoke may also be explained by tar, heavy metals, and other factors. Also, many of the aflatoxin-prone foods share other properties suspected in peanut allergy.

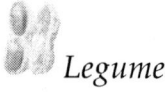
Legume

Charge: Substance.

Direct and corroborating evidence. Maybe. Typically, 10% or less of people with peanut allergy report allergy to other legumes.[94] Some commonly allergenic legumes, like soy and lentil, are among the most commonly and heavily consumed ones. Others, like lupine, are not.[95]

Motive: Yes. Legumes are botanically related. In Ayurveda, people who are encouraged to avoid or consume peanuts may or may not be told to do likewise with other legumes.

Exculpatory evidence: Yes. The legumes share many other suspect properties.[96]

Nut

Charge: Substance.

Direct and corroborating evidence: Maybe. Typically, 35 to 50% of people with peanut allergy self-report being allergic to one or more nuts.[97] I have not found a clinical study of people dosed with one sort of nut or another.

Motive: Maybe. Nuts come from various botanical families, some of which have many allergenic members (like the walnut-pecan family) and some of which have few to none (like the almond-plum-apricot-peach family). Tree nuts are not botanically related to peanuts.

Exculpatory evidence: Yes. The tree nuts share other suspect properties.[98] Peanut and nut allergies may be independent developments reflecting immune weakness.[99] Belief that tree nuts are related to peanuts may have an effect.

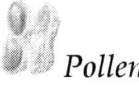*Pollen*

Charge: Substance.

Direct evidence: Maybe. Pollens can provoke anaphylaxis.[100] I have not found a study on peanut pollen specifically.

Corroborating evidence: Maybe. Some of the plants that yield allergenic foods have pollens that are allergenic – but not necessarily to the same people.[101] Pollen may be part of allergy to insect stings.[102]

Motive: Yes. Foods from a given botanical family may elicit a common, unique pollen-related IgE.[103]

Exculpatory evidence: Yes. These foods share other suspect properties.

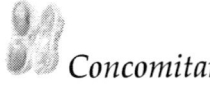*Concomitant pollen*

Charge: Substance.

Direct evidence: Yes. People who are allergic to pollens such as birch and grass may be more likely to be peanut-allergic.[104]

Corroborating evidence: Yes. The same is true of allergy to other foods. This includes those like nuts, fruit, and tubers that are closely related to the reproductive parts of plants, and those that aren't, like fish.[105]

Motive: Maybe. There may be some genetic similarity between allergenic pollens and unrelated, allergenic foods.[106]

Exculpatory evidence: Yes. Food allergies occur not just pollen season; I have not found information on how peanut allergy reports vary through the year.

Suitability to people

Charge: Pre-condition.

Direct and corroborating evidence: Yes. Allergy, asthma, eczema, hay fever, and other conditions cluster in families.[107] Peanut allergy is usually shared by identical twins, and is more commonly shared by siblings than by unrelated peers.[108] People who have different ethnicities, yet live in the same place and have similar lifestyles, can have very different rates of peanut allergy.[109] There may be a common genetic factor in allergies to the various legumes.[110]

Motive: Maybe. I have not found a finished study that identifies a peanut allergy gene, but research is in progress.[111]

Exculpatory evidence: Yes. Families share environmental, dietary, lifestyle, and other factors that may contribute to allergy.

Something about how peanuts are produced

Cotton pesticides

Charge: Substance.

Direct evidence: Maybe. The toxicity profiles of the most common US cotton pesticides, whether chemical (like paraquat, propargite, and methyl parathion) or biochemical (like *Bt, bacillus thuringiensis*), do not match anaphylaxis/allergy.[112] Neither do those of their impurities, like dioxin.[113]

Corroborating evidence: Yes. Corn, which is the other common crop in the peanut-cotton rotation, is a commonly reported allergen.

Motive: Maybe. Pesticides affect a host of organs and systems, some more directly involved in anaphylaxis/allergy and some less. For example, paraquat is a herbicide that sabotages weeds' ability to breathe and eat *(photosynthesize)*; in humans it irritates the mucus membranes of mouth, stomach, and intestine and damages the lungs, kidneys, liver, and heart.[114] Few to none of these studies cover long-term, low-level exposure.

Exculpatory evidence: Yes. Pesticides cause irritations and other symptoms that may be mistaken for allergy. Corn has some of the other properties (like intensive breeding) suspected in peanut allergy.

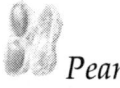 *Peanut pesticides*

Charge: Substance.

Direct evidence: Maybe. Common US peanut insecticides, herbicides, fungicides, and nematicides, like aldicarb, phorate, 2,4-D, chlorothalonil, and 1,3-dichloropropene, do not match the peanut toxicity profile.[115]

Corroborating evidence: Maybe. Some of these are used on other allergenic plants and some aren't. Meanwhile, each of those plants can have pesticides not used on peanuts.

Motive: Maybe, as with the first comment about cotton pesticides.

Exculpatory evidence: Yes, as with cotton pesticides.

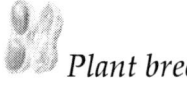 *Plant breeding*

Charge: Substance.

Direct evidence: Maybe. I have not found a study comparing the allergenicity of peanut cultivars of today and yesterday.

Corroborating evidence: Maybe. Many common allergens (like soy, eggs, cow's milk, wheat, and corn) come from heavily bred plants or animals; some (like white fish) do not. Switching to a less bred relative (like sheep's or goat's milk) can ease or eliminate allergy. Among crops that may be grown from genetically modified stock (in the US, these are beet, canola, corn, flax, papaya, potato, rice, soy, squash, and tomato) there are allergens and non-allergens.[116]

Motive: Maybe. Different peanut cultivars have significantly different levels of aflatoxin, but not necessarily of allergenic proteins.[117] The amino acid profile of their proteins and the fatty acid profile of their fats vary.[118] Low aflatoxin, high oil, high protein, and high vitamin varieties have been bred, but I have not found a study on how this affects allergy in the event that they have been introduced commercially.[119] Genetic modifications are also being tried, for example to boost vitamin A or to lower allergenicity, but these peanuts are not yet licensed for market.

Exculpatory evidence: Yes. Intensive breeding tends to target foods that are also intensively farmed, refined, and consumed – each, a possible factor in the incidence of allergy. The choice of cultivar has to do with climate, soil, and other factors, each of which in turn can affect protein, aflatoxin, and other suspect properties.[120] Some of the genetically modified cultivars licensed for growing may not yet actually be on the market.

Something about how peanuts are consumed

Form and amount

Charge: Substance.

Direct evidence: Maybe. I have not found a study on how a given person can respond differently to different prepared forms of peanut. There are studies on how a group of people responds to one form – many on dry roasted whole nuts and peanut butter and few or none on peanut sprouts and irradiated peanuts, for example.[121] I have not found a study on the incidence of allergy versus the amount and form of peanuts consumed daily.

Corroborating evidence: Yes. Most of the commonly reported allergens, like nuts, eggs, milk, soy, and some fish and shellfish, are being consumed in forms and amounts unprecedented for those people. I have not found studies on incidence versus form and amount. Transgenic forms may have an added problem: the splicing of one species' genes into another's (for example brazil nut into soy) can provoke allergy in people who are allergic to one but not normally the other.[122] Non-traditional diets have been associated with higher rates of asthma.[123]

Motive: Yes. How peanuts are grown and/or prepared affects many suspect properties.[124] More peanuts means more aflatoxin, protein, arachidonic acid, pollen or other problem substance, though this does not necessarily imply stronger effects.[125] It may also mean that people who would not normally choose to eat peanuts are eating them as hidden ingredients in packaged and served food. There are many examples of reactions to new foods or foods suddenly eaten in large amount: addiction and diabetes among Native Americans exposed to alcohol and refined carbohydrates; heart system clogging and disease among people who eat a lot of cholesterol and trans fatty acids from industrially hydrogenated oils; and so on.

Exculpatory evidence: Yes. It could be that, as more people eat more of a food, reactions are reported more often and the spectrum of effects widens. A person's perception of novel foods, for example those from another culture or that have been genetically modified, may affect their reaction.[126]

Previous exposure

Charge: Pre-condition.

Direct evidence: Maybe. I have not found a study of the frequency or severity of peanut allergy in people as related to the timing or level of first and later exposures. Anaphylaxis can occur without previous known exposure.[127] In a group of children followed from age one to age ten, overall, reaction worsened slightly.[128] Lab mice may react more strongly to eating peanut protein if they have been exposed earlier, through the skin.[129] They may react worse after a low prep dose than a high one.[130]

Corroborating evidence: Maybe. I have not found such studies on other allergens.

Motive: Maybe. Once a person is exposed to an allergen, they would develop IgE specific to that food. Some studies on peanuts and other foods show that high allergen-specific IgE makes a person more likely to become allergic to that food, while other studies do not.[131] On the other hand, once a person has developed the allergy and then outgrown it, continued exposure may keep it from coming back.[132] IgE levels may not be different in people who have and haven't outgrown peanut allergy.[133]

Exculpatory evidence: Yes. The emotional effects of prior exposure may not be separable from the physical ones. How a person reports their allergy may change as they get to know and articulate themselves.[134]

Exposure in the womb

Charge: Pre-condition.

Direct evidence: Maybe. In one study, the more peanuts mothers reported having eating while pregnant or nursing, the younger their children became allergic, if they did so at all.[135] I have not found a study tracking actual exposures. Avoiding peanuts while pregnant does not prevent allergy in children.[136]

Corroborating evidence: Maybe. I haven't found follow-up studies on the children of mothers consuming other allergenic foods.

Motive: Yes. Peanut aflatoxin, protein, and phenols can all cross the placenta, from mother to infant.[137] A mother's exposure to aflatoxin may increase the risk of birth defects, in general.[138]

Exculpatory evidence: Yes. Given the risk of harming pregnant women and their fetuses, here we have to rely on retrospective self-reporting, rather than deliberate dosing and monitoring.

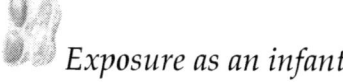 *Exposure as an infant*

Charge: Pre-condition.

Direct evidence: Maybe. In some studies, exposure to peanut as an infant makes a person more likely to become allergic then or later; in others, it doesn't.[139] It has even been proposed that early exposure may build tolerance.[140]

Corroborating evidence: Maybe. As with peanuts, infant exposure to food and non-food allergens may favour, prevent, or have no bearing on later allergy.[141]

Motive: Yes. A mother who eats peanuts can have the protein come out in her breast milk.[142] Food aflatoxin also appears in breast milk.[143] Allergy and asthma are related to faulty development of the immune system early in life.[144] A baseline condition of asthma can favour the development of peanut allergy.[145]

Exculpatory evidence: Yes. Early direct exposure to peanuts implies absent or limited breastfeeding. This can damage the immune system and imply the infant is more exposed to allergens in formula, cow's milk, and other foods, including peanut.

Something about lifestyle

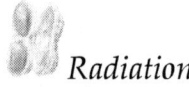 *Radiation*

Charge: Pre-condition.

Direct evidence: Maybe. I have not found a study on how exposure to radiation relates to the incidence of peanut allergy.

Corroborating evidence: Maybe. I haven't found one for other allergies, either.

Motive: Yes. Chronic or freak exposure to any of the high-energy forms of radiation can injure or kill immune and other cells and provoke diseases of many systems and organs.[146] Cellular and systemic effects are also seen with all of the low-energy forms. Recent intensification of UV exposure due to ozone depletion is linked to immune system depression.[147]

Exculpatory evidence: Yes. Radiation can affect many other body systems, and so provoke a spectrum of symptoms that may overlap with those of food allergy.

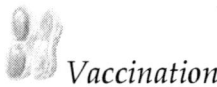 *Vaccination*

Charge: Pre-condition.

Direct evidence: Maybe. I have not found a study on the vaccination history of peanut-allergic and -immune people.

Corroborating evidence: Yes. Children vaccinated against tetanus (alone or with diphtheria and pertussis) can have higher rates of asthma and non-food allergy than unvaccinated peers. Measles-mumps-rubella vaccine has been linked to skin allergies. Pertussis and *bacille calmette guérin* vaccines may have no effect.[148] Multiple vaccination, as a whole, may lead to higher allergy rates.[149] I haven't found studies on the vaccination histories of people with various food allergies.

Motive: Maybe. I haven't found information on allergy-specific IgE in vaccinated versus unvaccinated people. Many human and animal studies of total IgE suggest it's comparable or lower in vaccinated subjects.[150]

Exculpatory evidence: Yes. Vaccines may contain allergenic proteins, as residues of the medium in which they are grown.[151] Side-ingredients *(adjuvants)* based on the metals mercury (like *thimerosal*, used in some measles-mumps-rubella vaccines) and aluminum (as in some diphtheria-tetanus-pertussis vaccines), have been blamed for increasing allergy and autism.[152]

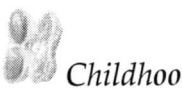 *Childhood illness*

Charge: Pre-condition.

Direct evidence: Maybe. I haven't found a study on the incidence of peanut allergy versus childhood disease history.

Corroborating evidence: Maybe. No information on other food allergies, either. Asthma may rise with early infection of the upper respiratory tract, but may drop or stay the same following other infections early in life.[153]

Motive: Maybe. The kind and amount of living toxins *(microbes)* to which a person is exposed can affect how their immune system develops and acts, but not always for the worse.[154]

Exculpatory evidence: Yes. The incidence of childhood illness has to do with sanitization, pollution, nutrition, emotional stress, family size, and other factors suspected in peanut allergy.[155]

Cow's milk and formula

Charge: Substance and pre-condition.

Direct evidence: Yes. Infants fed cow's milk or soy-based formula can be more likely to develop peanut allergy.[156]

Corroborating evidence: Yes. Infants who are exclusively breastfed have lower rates of allergy and other immune disease.[157]

Motive: Yes. Both soy and cow's milk contain allergenic proteins and aflatoxin.[158] Some infants who are allergic to cow's milk are not allergic to other animal milks, and some are. The same is true of children and adults.[159]

Exculpatory evidence: Yes. Cow's milk can contain hormones, antibiotics, and other substances that affect development and health. Its fat molecules are harder to digest than those found in milk from other farm animals and from humans.[160] Unlike human milk, it is typically consumed pasteurized, which may change how the body perceives it or prevent the immune system from learning how to deal with its microbes. Formula can contain sugar, preservatives, and other additives with health effects.

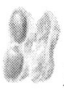*Pollution*

Charge: Substance and pre-condition.

Direct evidence: Maybe. I have not found a study of peanut allergy rates in areas of low versus high air, water, or other pollution.

Corroborating evidence: Yes. I haven't found studies on other food allergens, but non-food allergy and IgE may be higher in urban versus rural and high- versus low-traffic areas.[161]

Motive: Yes. Many common allergens, such as animal secretions, aflatoxin, and pollen, are borne by air and/or water.

Exculpatory evidence: Yes. Pollution refers to a whole array of substances, each of which may have various health effects.[162]

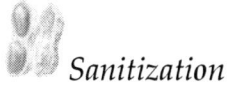 *Sanitization*

Charge: Pre-condition.

Direct evidence: Maybe. I haven't found a study on the incidence of peanut allergy versus exposure to dirt, sewage, and so on. The allergy is more reported in the developed world, where many traditional filth-borne diseases (like cholera, plague, polio, and typhoid) have been curbed by sanitization, vaccination, and other measures; while others (like e. coli, listeria, and salmonella) may have fallen, risen, or remain constant.

Corroborating evidence: Yes. Allergy rates may be higher among people who grow up less exposed to toxic bacteria and viruses.[163] I have not found studies on specific food allergens.

Motive: Yes. Allergenic IgE involves the same parts of the immune system that respond to some parasites, such as worms.[164] As discussed for the childhood illness theory, biological and other aspects of the environment affect immune system development.

Exculpatory evidence: Yes. Increased sanitization coincides with major changes to lifestyle and agriculture, any of which may affect allergy.

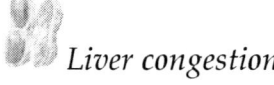 *Liver congestion*

Charge: Pre-condition.

Direct evidence: Maybe. I have not found a study on the comparative liver health or rate of liver disease among people with and without peanut allergy.

Corroborating evidence: Maybe. I haven't found studies on other allergens, either. Many of the commonly reported food allergens (like cow's milk and nuts) fit the theories of whole-body clogging, discussed earlier; others (like fish and soy) do not. People can also be intolerant to other clogging substances, like synthetic fats.[165]

Motive: Maybe. Peanut-specific IgE can be found in the liver.[166] Peanut aflatoxin may provoke or worsen liver diseases such as cirrhosis and cancer.[167] There may be a relationship to leaky gut.[168]

Exculpatory evidence: Yes. Clogging foods share many other suspect properties.

Leaky gut

Charge: Pre-condition.

Direct evidence: Maybe. I haven't found measurements of intestinal permeability differences between people with and without peanut allergy.

Corroborating evidence: Yes. Leaky gut has been found with allergy to foods such as cow's milk.[169]

Motive: Yes. Allergens cross the incompletely developed gut lining in infants, including those with allergies.[170]

Exculpatory evidence: Yes. There is a debate as to whether intestinal permeability is a cause or a symptom of allergy.[171]

Emotion

Charge: Pre-condition.

Direct evidence: Yes. People have psychosomatic reactions to peanuts.[172]

Corroborating evidence: Yes. Emotional allergies and intolerances to other foods and substances, like insect stings, are also documented.[173]

Motive: Yes. Feelings can alter the digestion and metabolism of foods.[174] Emotions such as depression and stress may or may not raise a person's IgE level.[175]

Exculpatory evidence: No. This is why it's controversial to admit emotions as a possible cause of peanut allergy: they can be used to explain or justify almost any finding or theory.

More Experiments

I just had a guest from the Philippines who said her countryfolk often eat peanuts boiled in shell. So I take out a couple more of those seed peanuts…

The shells smell like dirt or mold, not particularly appealing. I simmer them for half an hour, then remove the shells. The peanuts don't smell as good anymore, though not like bad smell-memories (say, of peanut butter cookies), either. As I'm about to take a bite, the phone rings. It's Mom. It's a sensitive moment to begin with, and her voice reminds me of comfort and panic. If only she knew what I was about to do… We talk, and then I need a minute to calm down.

It's not even that I particularly felt like eating peanut today. Sometimes of late I actually have. It's just, I wanted to keep progressing.

I chew off a small piece. It tastes a lot like sesame and a little like "bad peanut." Soon, my lips react. I spit it out. In my pocket are diphenhydramine (a reliable antidote) and milk thistle seeds (which sometimes work). I take some milk thistle. The reaction fades.

A few minutes later, I have some oatmeal, with another piece of peanut. I chew well and swallow. My lips tingle. I worry. Soon my chest and throat feel a bit irritated. I worry and feel safe. The reaction passes. Does that mean I can handle even more? That might be pushing it. Enough for today.

I've pushed myself a lot with allergy and life, blaming myself when things go wrong and feeling superior when they go right. Now it seems reaction and illness depend not only on things I'm aware of and control.

Another day, time to try a boiled, skinless peanut. This time, remove the shell before cooking. They're beautiful: full of life, safe. So why cook them?

I simmer some and nibble another one raw with breakfast. It reminds me of fresh peas and sprouted peanuts, pleasantly, with a trace of bad peanut. My mouth and system accept it. The boiled ones now seem faded, bloated, and unappetizing by comparison, and I don't try them.

A few minutes later I eat a bigger piece, maybe an eighth or quarter of a peanut. I didn't want this second bite as much as the first one. Soon there's a mild bad feeling in my mouth. Maybe I should eat something else. Maybe it was eating that second piece all by itself that's the problem. I fire up the corn popper. It's been one of my favourite foods lately. In a moment I'm starting to take gravely it reminds me of fun. As I wait for it to be ready, I grab my medicine but don't eat any. I think of all those times I was having a reaction and someone said, "maybe you should eat something else," and I'd say, "you don't understand, it doesn't work that way." Just smelling the popcorn and knowing it's coming, reaction and I calm down. Then I eat some and feel even better. Two hours pass without a problem. I guess all those people were right about something. And it doesn't even matter if it was for the "right reason."

I finally sowed some of those peanuts, a couple of weeks ago, in a pot indoors. Today I want to eat one of the sprouts. It smells and tastes good – fresh, alive, and new, like other sprouts, with no hint of bad peanut or various raw or cooked legumes, seeds, and nuts. It goes down good too. My first healthy, whole peanut! At least as far as I know.

The amputated sprout grows back. I dig out the skin of the peanut that made it, and rub it on my forearm. For good scientific measure, I rub the other forearm with a rough bit of another plant. Then I dust off the skin and eat it. In a few minutes, there's a big hive on the skin-brushed forearm and none on the other one, with maybe a little itch in my throat.

I run out of seed peanuts and go to the store to replace them. All that's available unroasted is non-organic ones, for eating. They sprout fine and go down so-so. At a certain point they stop growing and start developing a bluish mold. I don't want to eat any more.

I'm just sitting down to breakfast when I get in a fight with my landlord/friend and I was looking forward to calling Dad but his phone's busy. The food's a ridiculous combination with sprouted peanut and then Mom calls, we lock horns and wind up laughing. Pack my swim stuff and racquet not sure I should (can bring on strong reaction), start walking, call Dad, eat more crackers, work, eat, walk, nap, hear from another sometimes too-close friend watch tennis play tennis come for drinks? sure! then walk home underdressed tired write this feel fine.

The Full Medical

Age: 37

Sex: Male

Medication taken regularly: None.

Diseases or allergies: Allergy to peanuts and mold often and to some legumes and cigarette smoke occasionally. Intolerance to cow's milk as a child, with history of avoidance as an adult. Possible allergy to other foods or substances as a child. Strong positive RAST results to peanut and other extracts, up until teenagedom, with no testing since.

Ancestry and infancy. Eastern European Jewish. Immigration to Canada was mostly in grandparents' generation. For many generations, lifestyle seems to have been relatively urban, sedentary, and based on intellectual trades, with diet based on animal products, carbohydrates, and cooked vegetables.

Maternal great-grandmother reportedly died of asthma. Maternal grandfather's family had rampant heart disease and some asthma too. Paternal grandmother had arthritis and Parkinson's disease. Father has arthritis, with no allergies; smoked moderately until I was about 10 years old. Mother is allergic to scallops; gallbladder was damaged by pregnancies, such that by the time of my birth she had difficulty digesting fats and was eating little of them; experienced a major conflict then as well and became quite underweight; began switching to health foods (more fresh produce, more whole grains, fewer chemicals, and so on); smoked for much of my life to age 13. Two brothers, both older, have no allergies; smoked for many years.

History of allergic reaction. Two to three hundred reactions to date: most mild; 10 to 20 severe; at least 2 possibly fatal without medication, including first known reaction at age two.

Grade of reaction	Symptoms	Level of dose that caused it[176]
Zero	None	None or Low
Mild	Itchy lips and/or throat Concern Anxiety	None, Low, or High
Moderate	(any of the above, plus:) Swollen lips, throat, and/or eyes Difficulty breathing Hives, especially near lymph nodes (wrist, elbow, back, neck, groin); these swell when scratched Vomiting Gas and diarrhea	None, Low, or High
Anaphylactic	(any of the above, plus:) Suffocation Heart palpitation Panic	None, Low, or High

Course of a typical reaction. One or more waves, as follows. The strongest one is usually the 2nd, sometimes the 1st or 3rd.

Wave number	Time elapsed[177]	Grade of reaction	Level of dose	Type of dose[178]
1st	0 minutes	Zero to Mild	None, Low, or High	Local
2nd	15-45 minutes	Zero to Moderate	None, Low, or High	Local or Systemic
		Anaphylactic	Low or High	Systemic
3rd	2-3 hours	Zero to Moderate	None, Low, or High	Local or Systemic
		Anaphylactic	Low or High	Systemic
4th	6-8 hours	Zero to Moderate	None, Low, or High	Local or Systemic
		Anaphylactic	Low or High	Systemic
5th	24 hours	Zero to Moderate	None, Low, or High	Local or Systemic

The Sprouted Peanut Vaccine and Other Stories

Actions taken. In the following chart, success and failure are judged in terms of surviving a given wave and preventing or attenuating ensuing ones.

Grade of reaction	Successful actions	Failed actions
Mild	Doing nothing Calming self[179] Taking milk thistle[180] Taking diphenhydramine[181]	Doing nothing Calming self Taking milk thistle Taking diphenhydramine
Moderate	Calming self Taking milk thistle Taking diphenhydramine Taking epinephrine[182]	Calming self Taking milk thistle Taking diphenhydramine
Anaphylactic	Taking diphenhydramine Taking epinephrine	

Effects and side-effects of medication. Diphenhydramine becomes effective within 15-20 minutes and remains so for 2-4 hours. Staggered doses can prevent subsequent waves of reaction from being severe. It causes drowsiness and, when it wears off, leaves sinuses congested.

Epinephrine acts nearly immediately and lasts for 15-30 minutes. I used to carry Epipen but no longer do: it buys less safe time than diphenhydramine; diphenhydramine is usually strong enough; Epipen's expensive and expires quickly; as a hormone, I worry it can undermine rather than support my natural coping mechanism; and, as a powerful drug, I worry it can jolt me.[183]

If I eat a fair amount of peanut and reaction is moderate or strong, delaying medication makes anaphylaxis more likely. Strong reaction, especially combined with diphenhydramine or epinephrine, is usually followed by a day or two of exhaustion.

Milk thistle works often if taken as soon as mild symptoms appear but rarely if delayed until symptoms are strong. Using it with or in place of diphenhydramine often lowers or prevents congestion and exhaustion.

Role of food. Eating something starchy or sweet at the same time as peanut or soon after may prevent or reduce reaction. Eating something fatty or proteinaceous, especially of animal origin, may worsen it. Vegetables don't seem to have much effect.

Synthesis

For two months I've been living in a tent in the woods where it rains all the time. Everything's gone moldy. I'm having trouble breathing and can't get rid of it. Benadryl (diphenhydramine) is working but I worry I'll eventually become desensitized to it, and don't like the side effects. I wonder if there's an effective alternative.

For years I've been getting to know medicinal foods and herbs, using some to good effect. But this is a new situation. Better go ask the internet.

As usual, there's a whole variety of claims. Nettles and dandelions show up often. I've found those plants helpful before, as liver cleansers and blood tonics, and they happen to be growing nearby. Unfortunately, they don't work now. I wheeze on for a few more days and go back on-line to look up the history of diphenhydramine. I want to see if it's completely synthetic, or else if it or a similar substance can be extracted from a plant growing nearby or available from the herb shop in town.

The drug was first made in 1943, in the course of a search for antispasmodics. It didn't work so well for that, but the researcher, George Rieveschl Jr., was quick to realize what it was good for. Benadryl became the first commercially successful anti-histamine, and as recently as 2002 controlled 40% of the US non-prescription anti-histamine market.[184]

Next, I come across a newspaper article from 1999. "Arts patron and scientist George Rieveschl Jr. will be honored with the first presentation of the Cincinnati Art Museum's George Rieveschl Medal for Distinguished Service," it says.[185] That's only a couple of years ago! So – though he graduated from the University of Cincinnati in 1937, and would therefore be around 85 years old – there's a chance Mr. Rieveschl is still alive.

He is. In fact, he's now Vice-President of the University.

I call the main switchboard and ask for the VP's office. Once there: "Hi, is George in?" "One moment, I'll have a look."

"Hello?"

"Hello, Dr. Rieveschl, I'm a chemist with a peanut allergy, and I have a question about the experiment in which you discovered Benadryl. I would be grateful if you had a minute…"

He's gracious enough to have ten. Among other things, it turns out Benadryl is synthetic and he doesn't know of any plant connection. I thank him and sit back, amazed and somehow content that after all these years of searching, some of my illnesses and remedies defy perfect understanding or cure; that, from now on, in today's world, I'll carry milk thistle, Benadryl, and only the epinephrine that already runs in me.

The Peanut Detective Bod

"The Peanut Allergy Squad" was my attempt at an objective assessment of the peanut allergy theories. This chapter considers how they fit or don't fit my body's experience, and how that may bring new understandings.

Something natural about peanuts

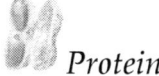 *Protein*

I react less to sprouted peanut than to unsprouted. Maybe it has to do with how proteins, starches, and fats change during sprouting; or with energetic or emotional factors, since sprouted peanuts smell, taste, and feel nothing like the forms of peanuts that remind me of danger. On the other hand, I have had little to no reaction to raw unsprouted peanut, whose proteins and other components are intact.

My experience with legumes is similar. I had had some reactions to them and understood their kinship to peanuts, so for many years I tended to avoid them. Eventually I started wanting to eat some, and sensed I could safely do so. I started with sprouts, which I'd read might be easiest to digest. They went down well, and I moved on to other forms.

It seems that, in general, having a lot of protein in my system, from any source, makes allergy more likely or strong. For example, during a recent spell of chronic exposure to mold, eating less protein significantly reduced my allergic symptoms.

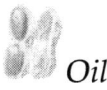 *Oil*

A few times, I have accidentally eaten peanut oil or chosen to cook with it. Usually there is no allergy, but sometimes for 2 or 3 days after I feel like I have a rock in my belly. So it may be hard for me to digest. This has been with refined peanut oil, which in principle would have little to no protein.

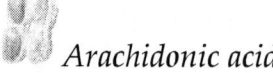 *Arachidonic acid*

I feel clogged eating a high arachidonic acid diet. I can't say whether this has to do with the arachidonic acid or with the proteins, fats, or other properties with which it comes. It alone doesn't make me have allergic reactions.

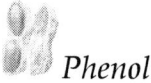 *Phenol*

I have no trouble with foods containing the same phenols as peanuts.

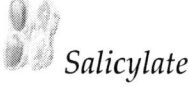 *Salicylate*

I have no trouble with most of the foods that contain salicylate, or with aspirin.

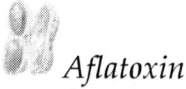 *Aflatoxin*

Chronic exposure to mold or cigarette smoke can give me similar symptoms to peanut allergy and anaphylaxis: tight chest and throat, asthma; heart palpitations; and panic; but not hives. Smelling cigarette smoke can make me instantly angry – even if no symptoms appear – and this used to happen with peanuts too. Even now that I can sometimes eat peanut, I can still react adversely to mold.

In one test, I got hives from rubbing a peanut's skin on my skin, but no reaction from ingesting the peanut's flesh. The skin may have more aflatoxin than the flesh, though a single test doesn't warrant much conclusion.[186] Meanwhile, I have often reacted to peanut butter, which is usually made from skinless peanuts.[187]

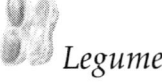 *Legume*

Lentils and split peas tend to give me a mild or moderate allergy, and maybe once gave anaphylaxis. Chickpeas sometimes give allergy, and once gave anaphylaxis. Soy and mung beans occasionally give mild allergy, but their sprouts do not. All other legumes are usually problem-free. Black beans are among my favourites.

I eat a little legume from time to time. They sometimes make me feel weighed down, and digest better at lunch than at breakfast or dinner. Other than sprouting, the way legumes are prepared doesn't seem to affect the chance of allergy or anaphylaxis. This includes methods reported to make them more digestible: using dried instead of canned; soaking and rinsing; cooking with seaweed or certain spices (such as fennel); and cooking without salt. I much prefer the taste and energy of legumes cooked from dry, after soaking and rinsing.

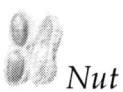 *Nut*

I have eaten all kinds of nuts, and not had an allergy or anaphylaxis that could be certainly blamed on them. I enjoy many nuts in small and occasional amounts, particularly almonds (historically) and walnuts and pecans (recently). Nut butters don't feel as good, and oils are so-so.

I understood that I should avoid nuts because of my allergy to peanuts. So I do have some fear about them. Sometimes when I'd have a reaction and didn't know what I'd eaten, I'd assume it was some nut and tell myself I had to avoid them. After many years, it didn't make sense that I should be allergic to hazelnuts, brazil nuts, and so on (I had even avoided coco"nut"); I wanted to try them and felt it would be safe. These were among my earliest, successful allergy experiments.

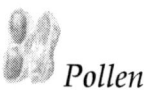 Pollen

Many of my allergies have been to legumes, whose pollens are related. I have not had problems with honey and other foods that may be particularly high in pollen. In general, I feel better eating leaf and root vegetables (which may be lower in pollen) than eating fruit and flower ones (which may be higher).

I often get congested in "allergy season" in the Spring. But I get the same symptoms in the Fall. So it may have more to do with the pattern of warm days, cool nights, and dampness. I have never had bad reactions to hay, grass, ragweed, or other plants, though they may contribute to those Spring allergies.

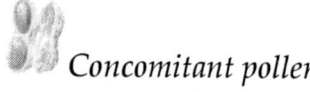 Concomitant pollen

I haven't noticed any seasonal pattern to the frequency or severity of my food allergies.

Suitability to people

There is a pattern of allergy, asthma, arthritis, and related conditions in my family. In Ayurvedic terms, I am predominantly vata and pitta, and have had particular trouble with peanuts and lentils, which people of both body types are recommended to avoid. My blood type is A, and peanuts and legumes are supposed to be good for us.[188]

Something about how peanuts are produced

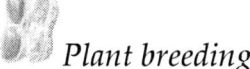
Peanut and cotton pesticides

I haven't noticed any allergy difference between foods that tend to be high in pesticides and those that tend to be low, or between a given food grown organically versus non-organically. The organic version often fills me up more and gives me more energy; if it's fresh – often, this means local rather than imported – I tend to prefer it too.

Plant breeding

Heavily bred and genetically modified foods don't seem to be any more allergenic than others. I'm not necessarily fond of their energy, which may also have to do with how they're grown and stored.

I wonder if the non-seed peanuts that stopped growing (in one of my experiments) had been altered in some way, say, by breeding, irradiation, or staleness.

Something about how peanuts are consumed

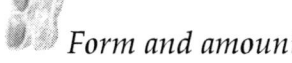
Form and amount

My ancestors come from a part of the world where, historically, peanuts were neither grown nor much eaten. They had some legumes, like lentils and split peas, and these are among the ones that have troubled me more. The sprouted and raw forms I find easiest to digest are not how they typically ate them. Other foods they probably didn't know – like subtropical fruit and grains, or goat and bison meat – tend to be problem-free or even among my favourites.

In general, the foods that feel best are whole grains, legumes, vegetables, fruit, and fish prepared simply. Many foods that come from more recent technology or fad – like white flour, nut butters, and solvent-extracted oils – don't feel good.

Suddenly eating a lot of any food that I tend to eat rarely or in small amount can be hard to take. It feels good to then go without it for at least a few days.

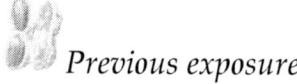 *Previous exposure*

Sometimes, I have mild reactions followed by strong ones, and sometimes the opposite is true. For example: after a mild reaction to some food contaminated with peanut, I had a strong reaction to its leftovers (that I thought weren't contaminated) two days later; another time, I had a strong reaction to chickpeas from one source and then no reaction to some from another source, two days later. In both cases, the fresher ones went down better. Other factors may have been time of day, mood, foods eaten at the same time, and, in the second case, ingredient quality and cooking method.

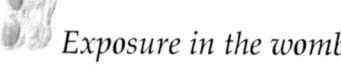 *Exposure in the womb*

My mother says she was fond of peanuts and probably consumed them regularly while pregnant with me. I don't know how to check if this had any bearing on my allergy. My brothers aren't allergic, and she likely ate peanuts while carrying them too.

Exposure as an infant

My first exposure to peanut was likely before birth. I don't know when I was first exposed out of the womb. My first strong reaction was at age two, which is within the timeframe some sources consider too young for giving peanuts to an infant. I don't know how to check if I would have reacted differently being older, or without having been exposed in the womb.

Something about lifestyle

Radiation

As far as I know, my mother and I weren't exposed to more radiation than our peers, though we may have gotten more than our ancestors. Radiation doesn't consciously bother me, though I dislike the feel of home and work environments with lots of electronics, and of microwaved food.

Vaccination

I was vaccinated against diphtheria, pertussis, and tetanus 5 times from age 3 months to 3 years, polio 4 times from age 3 months to 2 years, measles, mumps, and rubella once at age 1 year, and tuberculosis an unknown number of times starting at age 1 year. This was with the versions of the vaccines available in urban Canada in the early 1970s. I don't know how to check the relationship, if any, to my allergy, frequent colds and flus, and other childhood illnesses.

Recently, after many years with no vaccines and almost no prescription or nonprescription medicine, I had a bunch of shots in preparation for a trip to the tropics. I felt little or no short- or long-term effect, for example to immunity, energy level, or digestion.

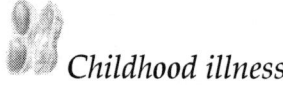 *Childhood illness*

I don't know if I had any big illness, whether common or unusual, before my first big peanut allergy. I seem to have had relatively fragile health as a child, with more colds and flus (and accidental injuries) than my brothers or schoolmates.

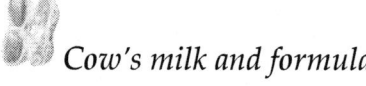 *Cow's milk and formula*

I was breastfed and never had formula, as far as I know. Cow's milk was introduced at some point; I was intolerant, perhaps with indigestion and fits. I have always disliked it and never chosen to drink it. The dairy product I did best with was yogurt. To this day, on the rare occasions that I eat it, I prefer fermented, unpasteurized goat's or sheep's dairy; this fits with theories about what's easiest to digest.

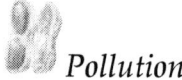 *Pollution*

I have lived mostly in a big city. In principle, then, I have had a relatively high exposure to certain kinds of pollution. I don't know how to check for any allergic effects. Smog and other summertime pollution can give me breathing trouble. Leaving the city clears it, and so does swimming underwater.

I haven't noticed any connection between the severity of an allergic reaction to a food and the pollution of my environment at the moment or in preceding days. But, when I feel internally polluted – clogged, emotionally overwhelmed, and so on – I am more picky and sensitive to the effects of my foods and environment.

Sanitization

Growing up in a good neighbourhood of a modern First-World city may also mean that I have had a relatively low dose of biological toxins. I haven't noticed any connection to allergy. I like a clean but not sterile environment, and fresh but not necessarily dirt-free foods, and have been mostly fine traveling in places with poor sanitation.

Liver congestion

In general, the things that supposedly clog one's liver don't make me feel good: eating past the point of fullness; snacking all day; eating rich for days on end; and so on. Sometimes then I will notice a pain or tightness in my liver-gallbladder area, and in the gallbladder meridians.[189] I feel restored to balance by eating less and simpler for a few days – particularly, less animal protein and fat.

Dairy, seed and nut butters, and fatty, grain-fed meat are among the foods that feel most clogging. They go down better in small amounts, at small meals, and especially with lemon juice, which in principle helps cut their fat and acidifying nature.[190]

Leaky gut

Intestinal problems, like constipation, have been some of the worst and most enduring of my life. Most of them I now attribute to stress.

The few times I get diarrhea and nausea tend to be: during a strong allergic reaction; after eating peanut without reaction; or with the flu. They feel like an attempt to reject something unwanted inside.

I haven't been able to feel anything as subtle as a change in my intestines' permeability, following one sort of meal versus another.

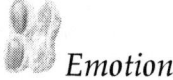 *Emotion*

Tasting or smelling peanuts has often agitated me. So has simply knowing they are present in the room. I've had severe allergic reactions merely dreaming of eating peanut. And I have sometimes had little or no reaction when choosing to eat peanut and attending to the resulting feelings.

So What Do You Think?

I'm curious.

About which of the theories presented so far are you interested to read more? On which do you think researchers should keep working? Do you have any big questions about the cause of peanut allergy, that none of the theories can answer?

If you wish to share your thoughts, you can e-mail me at the address inside the title page, and I'll send you a summary of everyone's input.

My Game Plan

How do I tell intolerance, allergy, and anaphylaxis apart, based only on symptoms?

Intolerance can be anything from a mild nuisance to a severe irritation; physical and/or emotional; instant or delayed; and not life-threatening. For example, most of the time, sugar and bread make me high and then sleepy, fried foods feel cloggy, caffeine withdrawal gives me headaches, chillies irritate my skin, and dusty air makes me cough.

Allergy is a mild or strong, systemic (therefore delayed), non-life-threatening response to an inert or living substance. Hence symptoms like heart palpitation and swollen lymph nodes. Once I've had such a reaction, I can reproduce it with or without exposure.

Anaphylaxis is an allergic reaction that develops rapidly and strongly enough to cross a threshold of whole-body panic. It can be life-threatening.

Intolerance and allergy may be absolute-sounding words for what is actually a continuum of knowing how foods and environments are better or worse for me.

Are all incidences of peanut anaphylaxis attributable to one cause, to which therefore anyone in that situation should be vulnerable?

Probably not.

Is there a set of factors that is always responsible?

Maybe.

Which causes seem most likely?

- ☆ Aflatoxin;
- ☆ Peanut protein;
- ☆ How these and/or other properties are affected by the way peanuts are grown, processed, and consumed – especially heavy breeding, partial hydrogenation, and rancidity from long storage after processing (shelling, skinning, hydrogenating, roasting, and/or pureeing);
- ☆ Emotions;
- ☆ An inherited potential to react that is greater than others';
- ☆ Faulty development and/or confused functioning of the immune and other systems – due to trauma, stress, pollution, sterilized food and environment, vaccines, nurturing with cow's milk or infant formula, malnutrition (from unbalanced diet and/or nutrient-poor food), and/or diet that is hard to metabolize (from pasteurized or stale ingredients, under- or over-cooking, combining incompatible foods or too many foods, eating too fast, too much, or too frequently, and/or heavy protein, fat, hormones, antibiotics, pesticides, or pollutants, especially from grain- or meat-fed animal products and bottom-feeder or carnivorous fish and shellfish);
- ☆ Certain foods, drugs, or other foreign substances, and/or their metabolites, present in the body at the moment of exposure to peanut.

Many of these factors can be changed, instantly or over time, by choice.

Could any one of these factors unleash anaphylaxis in a person?

Some yes, some maybe, some no.

How about a combination of them?

Yes.

Will it always do so in that person?

Probably not anaphylaxis, but maybe allergy.

Is there a way of understanding anaphylaxis holistically?

Yes. Many of the above factors seem to say parts of the same thing: allergy is a bad reaction to a normally good substance; it may come from inherited or lifestyle-induced damaged to immune and other systems; and if that substance has changed significantly, over decades or at some key moment, then it may no longer be good, and we may have a communication problem between body and food.

Given that altered and partly killed organisms are the bases of many vaccines, it is not surprising that refined, pasteurized, irradiated, and otherwise manipulated foods can trigger the immune system.

Does there have to be an anaphylactic substance?

No. There can be emotional reactions. These and more purely physical ones both feel like the momentary embodiment of major lifestyle and environment changes that have been happening for the past couple of generations, for many people, and with which, for whatever reason, I sometimes can't keep up. As food becomes richer, work more time-pressured, physical activity more polarized between being sedentary and working out, and rest less complete, body and feelings get overloaded, develop illnesses, and become sensitive to further intense stimulation.

Does this mean there is a universal way to prevent or weaken anaphylaxis?

Maybe. My experience is, if I can be allergic to something inside my body, in relationship with the environment, then I can also get to know it and change it. This may work for someone else in whole, in part, or not at all, and they may have their own special solutions.

Can the underlying problem simply resolve itself without being understood or acted upon?

Yes, as documented earlier.[191]

In summary, can peanut anaphylaxis be prevented with certainty, in any person?

Probably not.

Are some people more at risk than others?

Yes, given that some have anaphylaxis repeatedly and others never do.

Can a person reduce their risk?

Yes.

Can they eliminate it?

Maybe.

As someone who has had allergic or anaphylactic reaction to peanut, what have I done to prevent or attenuate future reaction?

- ☆ Avoid unchosen exposure to peanut;
- ☆ If exposure occurs, stay calm and take appropriate medicine, if needed;

- ☆ Keep the physical and emotional pre-conditions of allergy and anaphylaxis from accumulating, by maintaining digestion, elimination, detoxification, and other systems;
- ☆ Avoid mold and cigarette smoke, thus in principle aflatoxin;
- ☆ Try to find safe ways of getting used to peanuts.

How do I avoid peanuts?

- ☆ Cook from single ingredients (which also tends to be more appealing, nourishing, fun, and affordable);
- ☆ Read ingredients before buying packaged food and skip products that contain peanuts or "may contain peanuts," though not necessarily those labelled "may contain traces of peanuts;"
- ☆ Before buying ready-made food, ordering food, or receiving food: know from experience if it's likely to contain peanut; mention my allergy and see if the person understands; check ingredients and if they're sure; if peanuts are used in other dishes, verify that mine was or will be prepared and served with clean utensils.

Banning peanuts from an environment may protect me, but it can also give a false sense of security, since it's hard to enforce for sure. It's most important to tell people about the risk and check what I'm touching and eating when far from a medical facility that can treat anaphylaxis.

How do I unclog and nourish body and feelings?

In terms of everyday habits:

- ☆ Minimize foods containing synthetic or heavily refined ingredients;

- ☆ Moderate rich foods, which often means moderating protein and arachidonic acid;
- ☆ Have some more complex meals (like beans and brown rice) and some simpler ones (like crackers and fruit);
- ☆ Emphasize foods whose ingredients are naturally grown, recently harvested, unpasteurized, raw or moderately cooked, and simply combined, in other words full of live energy and enzymes;[192]
- ☆ Eat moderate portions, slowly, at rest, and with few distractions;
- ☆ Eat only when hungry;
- ☆ Generally, have at least three hours between meals or snacks;
- ☆ Once a week, skip a meal or fast for a whole day;
- ☆ Drink water regularly;
- ☆ Improve the quality of air breathed, in part by having outdoors time and keeping windows at least partly open;
- ☆ Improve drinking water;[193]
- ☆ Wash regularly and keep skin healthy (scrub well, moisturize when dry, clear when oily, and so on);
- ☆ Be active and rest well;
- ☆ Have at least a little time each day doing nothing, awake;
- ☆ Be with people and in surroundings that feel good;
- ☆ Have some alone, quiet time;
- ☆ Practice containing and expressing, privately or in an appropriate public way, the whole range of feelings I can have, including ones (like desire and anger) that may be taboo in many contexts;
- ☆ Work though feelings about illness, allergy, and peanuts;

- ☆ Practice staying calm and functional in stressful situations;
- ☆ Reduce chronic stress;
- ☆ Have support and advice;
- ☆ Practice sustained pleasure;[194]
- ☆ Minimize substances that may be poisonous and/or make it harder to feel how I am, and so allow illness to set in when I could be nipping it in the bud (for example, refined and artificial sweeteners, coffee, tea, energy drinks and bars, alcohol, cigarettes, marijuana, sleep aids, headache pills, laxatives, and stomach upset medicine);

Periodically I can do a more intensive cleanse and tone:

- ☆ Rest more;
- ☆ Work out more;
- ☆ Undereat a bit at every meal, for a few days, or fast for a day or two;
- ☆ Add rich but unclogging foods like seaweed, *miso* (fermented soybean paste), or liver;[195]
- ☆ Add fresh lemon or lime juice to water or food;[196]
- ☆ Drink more water;
- ☆ Tone done my environment (listen to music less often or more quietly, read less, watch less TV and movies, sit at the computer less, have low light or only natural light sometimes, be with fewer and/or less intense people, and so on).

Many of these things make it easier to eat some "unhealthy" food that just tastes good or that I want to share. I can be so health-conscious that it spoils my mood and social life. Here's part of the struggle with having known what it's like to feel sort-of sick all the time and really sick sometimes, and not wanting to go back there.

The Sprouted Peanut Vaccine and Other Stories

At any moment in time, I can be clogged in some ways, deficient in others, and functioning easily in still others. Clogged conditions like to be stripped down; deficient ones, to be built up; all, to keep neutral habits. When a problem comes up, I can look at the symptom for clues to the cause and remedy. For example: "nothing's going down and I'm not hungry" (clogged, so eat simpler); or "I'm stuffing my face and still not satisfied" (deficient, so eat richer). If I go overboard treating it I may get other weird symptoms, like the aggression or despair that can come from too-fast detox. I'll also eventually notice if I'm sticking with the adjustment after it's no longer needed: say, I feel fine but keep losing or gaining weight. That said, a certain amount of "stuff coming up" is part of the healing process, and some new habits stick, for the better.

What hasn't worked or seemed necessary?

Supplementing vitamins, minerals, and other substances (B_{12}, C, iron, glucosamine, and so on), even with their co-factors for assimilation, doesn't seem to do much. It feels better – more effective, fewer side-effects, less risk of creating a new imbalance – to instead present my body with a naturally balanced matrix (like unrefined sea salt or food grown in rich soil) from which it can pick and choose what it needs.

In a similar way, exercise, rest, hydration, and modest eating let me get rid of whatever I need to, more selectively and gently than enemas, chelation therapy, or long fasts, for example.

Once a year, I go for a nutrition status blood test, just to check.

Can I change my allergy?

Maybe. Experimenting with legumes, including peanuts, sometimes reveals that I misunderstood my reaction, that it has changed, or that there are new and safer ways to prepare the food.

In the process, my body may get familiar enough with it to handle it differently.

Should I?

Only as long as I want to, sense that I can healthily do so, and take appropriate precautions. Though I can react strongly to eating a small amount of peanut, I am not sensitive to the point that breathing or eating a speck can kill me on the spot; if I were, I wouldn't experiment.[197]

How do I begin?

Ideally speaking:

- ☆ Check where I'm at in my attitude toward peanuts and how this relates to my outlook on life;
- ☆ If ready to make changes, let the impulse to try come from within, not from someone else's push (though their support can be helpful);
- ☆ Let the idea of what to try follow from that, not from someone else's recipe (though their experience can be instructive);
- ☆ Even if it surprises me, trust it, and rest assured that I'll go slowly and gently enough to know if it's working or needs to be adjusted or stopped;
- ☆ Choose one thing at a time and do it consistently, say, for a week or two, with time to rest between attempts, and without making any other major changes in the meantime;
- ☆ Don't expect results;
- ☆ Base "is it working?" on how I feel inside and am relating to people and environment;

- ☆ Be aware that sometimes healing means facing an illness more fully, so it may seem to get worse when that's actually part of it getting better.

As time goes on, I learn to distinguish the latter, beneficial kind of struggle from things that are simply unpleasant and unhealthy, and so don't need to be tried.

How do I do tests?

- ☆ Have medicine and a calm, competent support person on-hand;
- ☆ Be certainly within 15 minutes of a hospital or clinic that is open and has room;
- ☆ The first time, take a small amount of peanut, raw or sprouted, skinless, from a fresh supply, with some simple complementary food like oatmeal (cooked in water), on an empty stomach, with no intoxicants or pharmaceuticals in the system;[198]
- ☆ Then rest or be mildly active, and watch for signs of reaction, especially instantly, within 15-30 minutes, and within 2-3 hours;
- ☆ Deal with any reaction as best as known from experience, trying to avoid panic and over-medication;
- ☆ If there is no reaction or mild one, wait a week or more, then retry the same thing, and if that too succeeds wait at least another week before trying a little more of the same thing or a small amount of peanut in different form;
- ☆ If there is moderate reaction, wait a week or more and deal with the effects and feelings, then, if the positive outlook and will are still there, try a small amount of a different form and proceed as above;
- ☆ If there is anaphylaxis, do not try again.

The Sprouted Peanut Vaccine and Other Stories

What has this taught me about the process?

It may take days or years; succeed each time, some times but not others, or not at all. Even if peanuts come to seem safe, do not assume unknown exposures, high doses, or new forms are. There might come a day when I can be completely free to eat peanuts, and there might not.

The forms and progression help me approach peanut as a new food, free of negative past associations and in digestible form. I get to know it in manageable form and amount, so that later I may be able to handle other forms or amounts. In this way, it's like a vaccination combined with a non-placebo-controlled oral challenge; a low-tech version of experiments on protein hydrolysis or mutation. Sometimes it feels like revisiting infancy and weaning: creating a safe and small space in which to learn my nature and become confident enough with it to go out into the world, where I may discover other things or be changed. Altogether, I move from seeing myself, life, and even allergy as problems, to living.[199]

It's a journey with zig-zags, curves, and u-turns as well as straightaways. I can be thrown off by taking in too much information or sensation, thinking about it too much, rushing, waiting to be sure, trying to control it all, or putting it all in the hands of "the universe," and brought back by humour, adventure, support, patience, passion, and more.

For someone who has never had an anaphylactic sensitivity to peanut, is it possible to reduce the risk of developing one?

I believe so, and that some of these nutritional and emotional tools may help. The first step would be to consult a qualified health professional, such as an allergenist, who can review a person's responses to peanuts and other foods, check the family history for allergies and related conditions, do an allergy test, and follow up. There are comprehensive books on the subject.[200] The only reminders I would add are that: a positive skin-prick test result or history of allergies in the family does not necessarily mean someone will become allergic; a pessimistic assumption can become self-fulfilling prophecy; and a negative RAST result does not necessarily mean the person is safe from allergy.[201]

What if it's a fetus or baby?

As a man who hasn't raised babies, I'm not in a strong position to speak. From what I've studied, if a pregnant woman eats some peanut, that will not necessarily harm the fetus or make the child develop an allergy later.[202] However, an excess of peanut or other cloggy food may not be good for a fetus or infant, given that it takes time for their systems to reach full capacity and for a parent or caregiver to get to know their particular constitution. Again, there are professionals who can provide guidance based on up-to-date knowledge.

The Sprouted Peanut Vaccine and Other Stories

Two
Something Deeper?

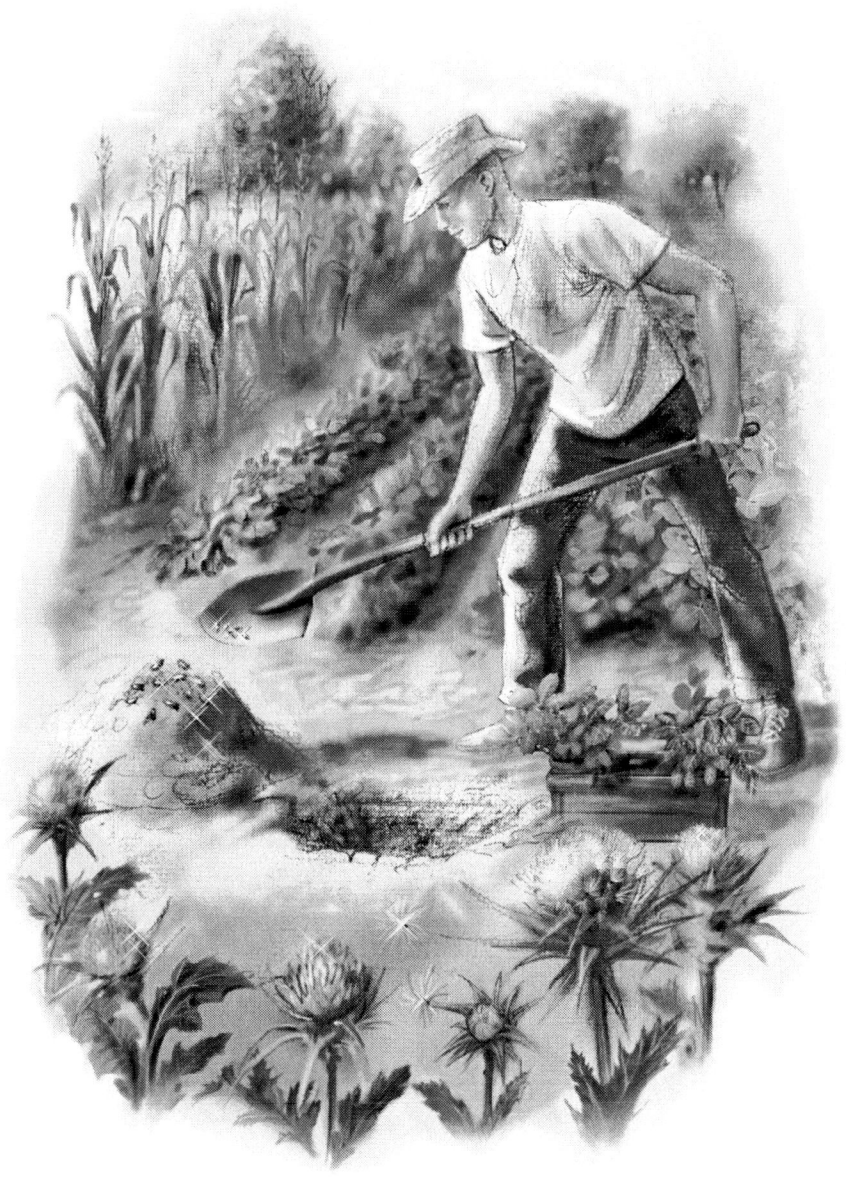

The Sprouted Peanut Vaccine and Other Stories

The Sprouted Peanut Vaccine and Other Stories

Related Symptoms

One day, I stumble upon a web page that makes some fascinating connections I can't include in "The Peanut Detective Squad," because there are no references and no information about the host organization. It describes a Dr. Klaus Wenzel's work treating people with allergy and other problems related to chronically high histamine levels. In twenty-five years of practice, he's found a particular cluster of symptoms:

- ☆ High histamine;
- ☆ Fast metabolism, often reflected in a lean body;
- ☆ Warm hands and feet;
- ☆ Abundant saliva, often leading to excellent teeth;
- ☆ Plentiful perspiration;
- ☆ High libido and easy orgasm;
- ☆ High sensitivity to pain;
- ☆ Stomach problems;
- ☆ Frequent colds and allergies;
- ☆ Chronic insomnia and below-average need for sleep;
- ☆ Low sensitivity to drugs and alcohol;
- ☆ Chronic depression, perfectionism, and/or overwork;
- ☆ Deficient chromium, manganese, zinc, and vitamin B_6.

To lower chronically high histamine, he recommends:

- ☆ Eating low-protein and mostly vegetarian;
- ☆ Avoiding refined sugar;
- ☆ Minimizing alcohol;
- ☆ Moderating folate intake;
- ☆ Monitoring chromium, manganese, zinc, and vitamin B_6, and supplementing as needed;
- ☆ Supplementing the amino acids glycine and/or methionine.

The host organization, Restore Unity, appears to be an advocacy or for-profit group in *orthomolecular* medicine.[203] I can't find much information on Dr. Wenzel, anywhere, in English; his German-language web site indicates a PhD in medicine and specialization in neurology and psychiatry.²⁰⁴ Various sites explain what orthomolecular medicine is about: supplementing deficiencies and purging excesses of vitamins, minerals, enzymes, amino acids, fats, and other substances already found in the body, without recourse to drugs, herbs, or non-essential nutrients.²⁰⁵ It doesn't seem to be well accepted by the medical community, but at least the supplementing aspect seems to be hitting the consumer mainstream of late.

The approach was defined by Linus Pauling, a chemist who around age forty was diagnosed with Bright's Disease – a kidney inflammation that impairs their ability to remove water-soluble toxins from blood – and reportedly told he was going to die. He went to see Dr. Thomas Addis, now known as one of the fathers of urine analysis. Addis prescribed a no-salt, low-protein, vitamin- and mineral-supplemented diet. Pauling lived another fifty years.²⁰⁶

I first heard of Linus Pauling as a champion of vitamin C, not knowing that's a small part of the orthomolecular story, or that he's one of only two people to win Nobel Prizes in different fields: Chemistry, in 1954 (at age 53), for developing our understanding of how substances are made from their atomic building blocks; and Peace, in 1962 (at age 61), for campaigning to stop above-ground nuclear testing.²⁰⁷

Also controversial, it seems, is Devi Nambudripad's approach, that allergy is the cause of 95% of illnesses and all can be cured with a mix of nutrition, acupuncture, chiropractic, muscle testing, and other methods.²⁰⁸ She has degrees in biology, acupuncture, and chiropractic, and her Allergy Elimination Techniques (NAET) are based on self-experiment followed by treatment of thousands of people. Today there are 9000 NAET practitioners worldwide, treating many times that population.

One of her students, Ellen Cutler, has developed a Bioenergetic Sensitivity and Enzyme Therapy (BioSET), using chiropractic, muscle testing, acupressure, and enzyme nutrition. From her perspective, peanut allergy/intolerance is related to asthma, attention deficit disorder, colon inflammation *(diverticulitis)*, depression, eczema, hyperactivity, recurrent ear infection, and troubled menopause.[209]

Harmony

I eat sprouted peanut and dream of singing.

We're thirty people in the basement of my childhood home. As a child, it's where I'd go watch TV after coming home from school, often to an empty house. If one brother or the other was around maybe we'd play ball hockey or something. How I hoped for those moments! When the brothers were together, I was often on the outside; I had some different needs and habits, like peanut allergy and being a morning person.

As a teen, my dad started being around more, and the basement became his second office and sort-of fitness area. On weekends, I'd wake up and go downstairs to hang out while he did his stretches and breathing exercises. His voice was softer and he was more accessible than usual. We'd talk for hours, first there and then over breakfast at one of our favourite places. Eventually, I started wanting to change things up – go to a different place, or do something else entirely. It was awkward. He liked the old habits. I didn't want to lose the connection. But I was changing fast – too fast, it has often seemed since, for the other person to keep up. Maybe if I'd heard of Wenzel I could have chalked it up to my allergic metabolism! Instead, I've been told and told myself relationships fail because I expect too much; people are scared by my initial expression of need or ultimate expression of disappointment.

The dream singing group's here for an improvisation workshop with the famous Bobby McFerrin. As if I'd long wanted to bring him to Montreal, and now here he is! I'm having trouble keeping up. The guys in the bass section are trying to help me learn our line and sing in harmony, but it's not working I'm distracted, getting down on myself, feeling not totally part of the group. Like it was as a kid, paddling, swimming, pedaling wildly, against a voice I hear to say, "you're not good enough, we're going to leave you behind."

I leave the room to go upstairs and see my brother. He's in the kitchen – Mom's domain. She's there, but out of sight, working on dinner. He's lounging in one of those 1970s space-age-looking chairs that used to live in the basement. I tell him, "what you said to me was abusive! It's about you, not me. Mind your own business!" I keep to myself the words, "maybe you too were hurt by someone, and that's how you learned to do this. I want you to heal yourself." There was always this conflict simmering just below the surface, and me fearing it would boil over; now it doesn't mind me removing the lid.

I go back downstairs. I'm sad to have missed part of the workshop and worried I may have lost my place. But, no, it's good I left to deal with that outside problem, for I'm readier to take the place that was there to begin with. The basses spread out to let me in, then close back tight around. It feels like an older brother laying his arm on my shoulder.

I'm eager to fit in, learn the songs, and sing! It's going to be a challenge. I was already behind and now have more catching up to do. The songs aren't easy and the group has begun to jell. As a kid, dad would help me catch up to or even get ahead of my brothers. Here I've got to do the work, and they're not going to hold me to any lower of a standard. I don't know if I can make it. I take big breath in. It doesn't block in my throat, but flows, out and in again. At first it sounds and fits so-so. The suggestions and instructions don't stop. Now I hear them as "we want you to get there, we need you." I pedal and paddle, sometimes even getting ahead, and then they catch up. I can sing! And do music, this music. From within its shell or scab a rich and nimble voice emerges.

In choirs, workgroups, and family, sometimes I almost yell, as if to prove I exist and matter. In this moment, you can barely hear me within the full volume and harmony.

Related Systems

In traditional Chinese medicine, health is dynamic balance between complementary kinds of energy: masculine (*yang*) and feminine (*ying*), hot and cold, interior and exterior, and excess and deficient. Each of these is used to characterize five elemental sets of body systems as they relate to each other and the environment:[210]

	Wood	**Fire**	**Earth**	**Metal**	**Water**
Organs	Liver Gallbladder	Heart Small intestine	Spleen Pancreas Stomach	Lungs Large intestine	Kidneys Adrenals Bladder Genitals Brain
Tissues	Tendons Ligaments	Arteries Veins Pericardium Chest, abdominal, and pelvic cavities	Muscles Flesh	Hair Nails Sinuses	Teeth Bones Nerves
Sense / organ	Sight / Eyes	Speech / Tongue	Taste / Mouth	Smell / Nose Touch / Skin	Hearing / Ears
Functions	Detoxify body Store and distribute nutrients Make mental and metabolic plans and decisions Maintain conscience Develop immunity	Adapt to environment Keep soul, mind, and feelings alert Maintain heart, circulation, thyroid, immunity, and lymph Protect organs of chest, abdomen, and pelvis and keep their fluids flowing Separate food from waste Make use of nutrients and information	Maintain digestive tubes and fluids Sustain reproduction and lactation Build and channel blood Hold organs in place	Eliminate stagnant energy Take in life-energy Regulate inputs and outputs	Cleanse blood Maintain vitality and adaptability Store excess energy Ensure survival and relaxation

The Sprouted Peanut Vaccine and Other Stories

	Wood	**Fire**	**Earth**	**Metal**	**Water**
Emotions	Anger Good nature Patience	Euphoria Hate Joy Laughter	Guilt Reflection Serenity Worry	Courage Depression Motivation Sadness	Fear Gentleness Nervousness Will
Taste	Sour	Bitter	Sweet	Pungent	Salty
Colour	Green	Red	Brown	White	Black-Blue
Climate	Windy	Hot	Damp	Dry	Cold
Peak season	Spring	Summer	Late summer	Fall	Winter
Rest season	Early Fall	Winter	Early spring	Spring	Summer
Peak time of day	Night	Early afternoon	Morning	Early morning	Afternoon-evening
Rest time of day	Morning-afternoon	Night	Evening	Late afternoon	Early morning
Animal life stage	Birth Infancy	Childhood	Adolescence Prime	Maturity	Old age Death
Plant life stage	Seed	Sprout Shoot	Flower Fruit	Seed	Dormancy
Farm year stage	Planning Sowing	Sprouting Weeding Thinning	Weeding Maintaining	Harvesting Celebrating	Processing Resting
Keyword	Direction	Passion	Grounding	Social life	Ancestry

In this sequence, each one feeds the next, as a parent. This *creative* cycle is balanced by a *control* cycle, whereby each element keeps the second-next in line, as a grandparent. When elements are left unchecked or imbalanced, they can overwhelm their grandparents, and reverse the control cycle into a *destructive* one. Symptoms appear, and the cause is sought. If a certain system is deficient, it can be supplemented using tonic foods and herbs or deep, slow massage, particularly during rest periods. If it is in excess, that can be broken down using reductive foods and herbs and vigorous massage, especially during peak periods. There tends to be a pattern of deficiency in some elements with excess in others, and the whole person gets treated. The theory gives some ideas, touch gives others, things are tried, responses are checked, and adjustments are made, until relative balance is restored.

Fire and Water

Dinner and dessert are great and I go to bed a little hyped. I'm tired but take a while to fall asleep. In the night I wake up thirsty. Drink, and still feel thirsty. Lay in bed a while, then get up to make sure the front door's locked. Come back to my room, curl an arm comfy over my crown, and sleep.

I dream it's dawn. An older man and a woman about my age are outside my room, playfully greeting each other and the day. Somehow my door is not solid wood anymore but windowed and curtained. They can peer at me, and do, and I don't mind. I'll join their fun when I get up.

Next dream, the man gets up and leaves my room – I didn't even know he was there to begin with. The woman enters and says, "I came to bring you your pillow." I'm about going to come, cover up, and do as she sits next to me, knitting.

I rent an apartment and have two roommates, one of each sex. We live separate lives. I've been getting annoyed with them because they don't seem to love me or this home the way I need, I feel left out of their club, and they don't seem to take my many requests – like locking the door – seriously.

For years I didn't lock the door, and even liked it when that surprised people. "What, you don't trust people?" I'd poke. Recently, in Benin, my host family insisted I lock my bedroom when leaving for the day. So did my host at the end of travel, six months later, in the United States. I got to like it. Earlier today I almost blew up at one of my roommates for not doing it. I'm confused. I want no boundaries in my home so that I have support blocking off the outside world. It doesn't seem to be working.

These wet and sweaty dreams tend to come in the early morning hours that Chinese medicine considers time for the bladder, kidney, and adrenal glands to rest, so that they can keep in line the volcanic fire of the heart and small intestine.

Unexpected Results

Not only is peanut reaction a shock; so is the fact that sometimes it's not, whether by choice or for reasons hard to understand or control.

I have tried to recall all of my surprisingly bad or mild reactions, to see if there's a pattern. As a reference point, the following table also gives some of the more important reactions that in retrospect would have been more predictable.

Strong reactions, even to low dose	Unexpectedly mild reactions to moderate or high dose
Age 2, home alone, with the nanny in the other room	Age 27, at the home of a girlfriend I loved and trusted and whose family I liked and felt accepted by
Ages 5 to 17, a few times, at school or camp; I'd tend to refuse help and go be alone	Age 30, at a restaurant with my parents
Age 19, at college, after playing squash with a guy I wanted to like me but didn't necessarily like	Age 33, twice choosing to eat sprouted peanut, alone
Age 20, visiting my brother at his college, after our parents had just left	Age 33, unknowingly eating peanut at a party at the home of a good friend and colleague
Age 29, at home, with a girlfriend I felt ambivalent toward, in part because she had a lot of negative feelings toward men	Age 34, eating chickpeas, alone, two days after having strongly reacted to them
Age 30, alone, eating leftovers of peanut-containing food from a restaurant, two days after having eaten them there with my parents	Ages 35-36, choosing to eat sprouted peanut, with my roommate around
Age 31, living in a moldy tent for two months	Ages 35-36, choosing to eat raw peanut, a few times alone and a few times with people around

The Sprouted Peanut Vaccine and Other Stories

Strong reactions, even to low dose	Unexpectedly mild reactions to moderate or high dose
Age 34, living in a new place (in West Africa), on a weekend when my main buddy was away	
Age 34, living in a new place (in North Africa), breathing lots of cigarette smoke every day	
Age 34, living in a new place (in Southern Europe), eating unfresh, unappetizing food, in this case chickpeas, with Jewish people, all of which reminded me of childhood experiences that felt stagnant and repulsive	
Age 34, living in a new place (in the US), right before my main friend, who felt like a father or brother, went away	
Age 35, on the first night living in a new apartment (in Montreal), with both roommates away, and a lot of mold around	

It seems that lack or feared lack of good-feeling male and/or female presence can worsen reaction, and that a balanced (masculine and feminine) quality of presence, from someone else or myself, can improve it.

Coming home from therapy

Sometimes it feels like Dad's pleading for something. Nourishment, and I try to give it to him, as if from my own flesh.

Mom likes to give us fancy cookware and produce. For a while I was into liver — curious to try a different kind of meat and thought I might need B_{12} and iron and it could give them. She still asks sometimes if I want some, from her organic butcher.

"Not today, thanks."

Unchosen Experiments

My first night in a new apartment, I'm having a hard time breathing and sleeping. Feels like a three-hundred-pound weight on my chest, like last year in Tunisia when everyone was puffing harsh cigarettes. Totally discouraged, can't imagine feeling good.

Wake up, find a bathroom full of mold. Roommates help clean up, health improves, though still puffy sinuses and tight breath sometimes. Then it comes back hard, and I want to flee my body, since I can't escape the mold. Reminds me of being a kid in a house full of smoke and tension, and who knows maybe mold too.

My roommate's smoking on the balcony and it blows inside and bugs me. Fifteen minutes ago I was at a party outdoors at someone else's home and folks were smoking and I was fine.

I've also been having sugar cravings, and headaches where I usually get them when in sugar withdrawal.

What is it about being invaded in my home – which begins with body and feelings – that can make me so intolerant?

The place I moved out of was my home for many years. At first it's owned by an elderly chiropractor and his wife. Then one day a slick guy rings and says I'm the new landlord, give me the rent, and are you Jewish? He must have noticed the *mezuzah* ornament blessing the doorway. I never know how to answer that question. Some people don't like Jews. Some think Jews are superior. Turns out he's Jewish. As for the rent, I say I've already paid and who are you? A couple of days later, a trip to city hall confirms the building's been sold to his numbered company.

Gene takes to hovering around the building, ringing people's doorbells, and trying to come in when we answer. The climate turns creepy and at times belligerent. One by one, tenants leave and rents are hiked. I'm the last to hang on. Things get worse. I'm sued for eviction, based on some dubious paperwork, and not sleeping so well.

I dream he lets himself in to show the place to a prospective tenant, and that wakes me up. I'm in the back and scared to face the intruder even though I know him. In my world male strength has often been equated with abusive violence; if I confront him, I risk being hurt (if I lose) or judged (if I win). I don't want him in my bedroom, but don't hurry to the front door, either. We meet in the kitchen. We have some words. I open a drawer, take out the chef's knife my mother gave for Christmas, contemplate it, and chase him through the apartment into the garden of my childhood home, where Mom and her girlfriends are having a tea party. The knife is in his back, and to my surprise they approve.

When my therapist asks, "what's a Nazi?" I say, "someone who tries to take your home away."

I'm trying to sleep, catch a whiff of smoke, and go knock on the other roommate's door. She's on the phone and doesn't answer. I knock again and finally she comes. "What is it?" "Are you smoking?" "No." Instant regret: I didn't respect her space or trust her to respect mine; worse, it showed. I wait for her to get off the phone and make pains to apologize. Feeling inept like the six-year-old who raged at family, teachers, or schoolmates for making noise when he was trying to sleep, or for not being careful about getting peanut on things. How to explain to them then, or my roommate now, why I act this way sometimes? If only I could stop shooting my relationships in the foot; if only I could make today the "tomorrow when everything'll be better."

Another time, far from mold and peanut, roommate or landlord, I struggle for breath the moment I sit down to tutor Chang. Sometimes I dread my work, with its intimate rapport and the demanding culture of science, but this isn't one of them. Chang's easy to teach, appreciative, and doing well. Mind you, what little he doesn't get, he gets worked up about.

A moment ago I was walking to meet him, with a smile on my face and a bounce in my step. I'd just polished off a big job and a pile of crackers and jam. Usually I keep my energy a little low. It makes it easier to handle food and feelings. Lately I've been feeling especially cleaned out. I like it but it makes me more sensitive.

I've always felt obligated to clean up or organize other people's litter, clutter, and feelings. It's what I grew up among, and with inside. Frankly, I can be intolerant to it – even allergic, it seems today. But watch me go clean up anyway, like a vacuum cleaner to the universe, with a fine filter that can suddenly go from super efficient to totally clogged and back again. Maybe other people can accumulate more or for longer before problems appear – but then have more to excavate when they do.

I've been easy to overwhelm and confuse and had to learn the boundaries of my body and feelings. As with any adjustment, sometimes I've gone far to the opposite extreme. Now it seems natural to feel at least some continuity with other people, not only in terms of the social or emotional but even in terms of our inner, physical nature and destiny. "No man is an island," so they say.[211]

I am fond of Chang and he bugs me. I was quick-witted and prone to tantrums too. It feels like that wild energy they talk about in biology: the lightning from above or volcanic heat from below that scrambled dead gases in air or minerals in water into living matter.

Hungry Foods

One reason I started checking if I was allergic to legumes, and if so if I could become unallergic, was my new vegetarian friends. They used a lot of them, and I wanted to share.

I developed a love of falafel – delicate, deep-fried balls of fava beans and/or chickpeas spiced with cumin and speckled with parsley. Strangely, when I'd eat some, even to excess, I'd wake up in the middle of the night craving more. Maybe there's some special nutrient it has that I'm missing, I thought. Maybe I'll have some more. Hm. The craving's still there, and I don't feel so good. It feels like how sugar, bread, pasta, and alcohol go down. These foods I associate with having a blast together but shamefully pigging out on alone.

From a student

Hi Adam, I have another question, if you don't mind. This question has actually been on my mind for a couple of years – I guess because it is an event that recurs through my digestive habits. Here goes:

Whenever I consume grains, especially in bread, I feel as though my stomach takes longer to feel full or satiated than when I consume legumes or vegetables, for instance. Is there a reason for why my stomach becomes, figuratively speaking, a bottomless pit when I eat grains as opposed to any other food group? Does this have something to do with the composition of the grains and how they interact with my digestive tract and my brain?

The Sprouted Peanut Vaccine and Other Stories

Three
From Death to Birth, Life, and Risk

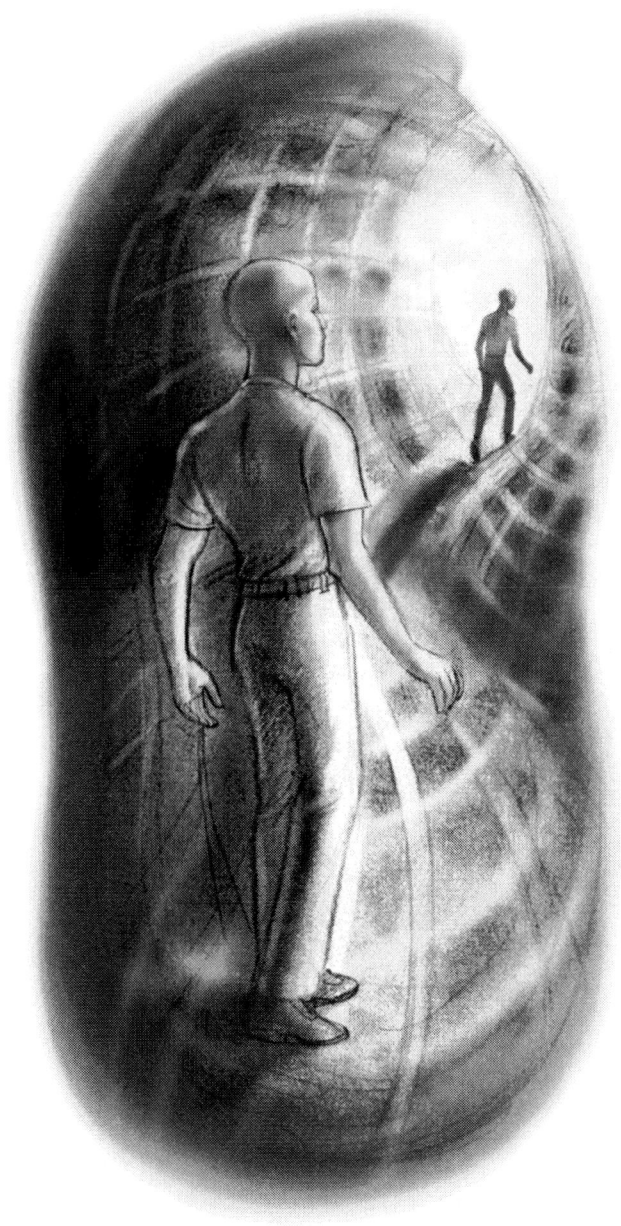

The Sprouted Peanut Vaccine and Other Stories

The Sprouted Peanut Vaccine and Other Stories

Our Child and Sibling

*A mother's experience of life with a child afflicted
with a peanut allergy*

Adam was 2 years old. Arriving home from work early, I was greeted with alarm by our housekeeper who had just proudly offered her freshly baked peanut butter cookies to the joy of her charge. To her shock, his face started to blow up and red blotches began to mark his body. He was beginning to have difficulty breathing. Panic overwhelmed. Called the pediatrician who urged me to get down to his office a.s.a.p. Called a taxi, sped down to the doctor with our suffering child who was by now projectile vomiting. Panic: were we going to lose him? Dr. R. assured us that we had just made it in time, for he was going into anaphylactic shock. "Thank God" for the adrenaline. Waited 45 minutes in the doctor's office. Things calmed down. We had our son back! That experience etched indelibly in my brain would foster a vigilance that would never leave me.

The doorbell rings. Girl Guides are selling their cookies. "Mommy I want one," enthuses 5 year-old Adam. Must find out what's in them. "Oh no, you can't have this honey, there may be peanut residues." A mother's relief tinged with sadness.

A birthday party invitation arrives. Better warn the parents. Come to think of it, better inform the school. But what about his friends who offer him treats at school or at their homes?

On holiday at Martha's Vineyard, we offer a treat of "M&M's." Little did we know that 45 minutes later we would be on the way to the hospital with our son, whose allergic symptoms were getting worse by the minute. Rescue and relief. From then on the Epipen was in our constant possession. How to instil an awareness of the seriousness of the risk and the precautions needed, without instilling a fear of living and a sense of vulnerability that would hamper his enjoyment of life?

As if he knew he had almost died on that first experience, as if he sensed the fragility of life, Adam acceded readily to all the constraints we imposed. "Let Mommy or Daddy read the label." "Don't eat anything anyone offers you without checking as to what it contains." "If in doubt throw it out!" was our motto.

As the teen-age years approached, sensing the importance of the need for autonomy, to feel competent and strong, there was my fear that feelings of vulnerability and fear might trammel his growth of confidence in himself and in life. Would he need to minimize the seriousness of the affliction? Would the need to be ever vigilant hamper his spontaneity? Although reaching out with support and understanding, I had to accept that he would chart his course in his own way.

What it's like to have a son with a peanut allergy

The first time I discovered that Adam had a peanut allergy was in Providence, Rhode Island during a Chinese meal. Suddenly, Adam had trouble breathing and we had to rush him to the hospital to save his life through an injection of adrenaline. That scared the hell out of me – as well as realizing that at any time in the future he would face a similar episode – I think Adam's parents were more frightened than he was.

While Adam has taken precautions since then, he doesn't want us monitoring his eating. It is difficult for me to say nothing when we go to a restaurant – he gets upset at being "babied." Lately, he has expressed the view that his allergy is "under control" if not "cured." I have told him that I find his attitude cavalier. Which he did not appreciate. What am I to do? I love him deeply and yet, I have to let him live his life as he sees fit even if it means taking risks.

Dear brother Adam

As a kid, I think your allergy to peanuts appeared to me mostly as a sudden interruption. Before I could grasp the fatality of it (or really understand the idea of fatality) it seemed to be something that erupted without warning, with the result that time immediately slowed down and everyone got very serious. Whatever fun we were having changed to intently watching your cheeks for creeping redness and swelling, and listening for the telltale wheezing that meant that your airway was narrowing. I suppose that part did resonate with me – I think that every active kid has the experience of being out of breath, winded, or starved for breath (as when you're on the bottom of the football scrum), so the panic of asphyxiation was somehow more comprehensible. I can't remember clearly who would panic more: you or the nearby "responsible adult" (mom, dad, a teacher, etc.). I think you were pretty scared, and that made me scared too. I don't think I saw you as fragile – it was just that something that I could eat without a problem was very poisonous to you. At the time, I didn't know anyone else who was so allergic to something. I felt bad that you had that particular added risk to deal with, but didn't understand why it was only you. I still don't – perhaps your thorough research and inquiry will shed some light on it.

I remember clearly the time you came to visit me when I was away at university in Providence, and how you got a reaction shortly after I took us to a Cambodian/Thai restaurant which I really liked, and had wanted to share with you. It was a pretty strong reaction, judging by how quickly you moved through the typical symptoms. At first I was mostly concerned with getting you to treatment as fast as possible, and then figuring out the logistics of how to pay the costs of that treatment (this was the U.S. after all), as I was now the closest thing to a "responsible adult" around. Once you were being cared for at the hospital, I could take the time to triple-guess myself and seek blame for your predicament. As your older brother, I certainly felt responsible for your being sick. I think that for a while afterwards, I was very reticent to eat with you at restaurants where your allergy couldn't be clearly communicated to the waiter or owner, and this ruled out adventuring to the newest ethnic food novelty, the pursuit of which is such a focus in cosmopolitan cities like Montreal. The risk was that such restaurants were often run by very recent immigrants, whose grasp of English of French was unreliable. I guess that the experience in Providence, and my/our evident and frustrating inability to communicate the seriousness of your allergy to the restaurant people, pushed me to seek safer choices when we were together.

When you got a bit older, you started to resent being singled out, being made obviously different, by mom, dad, me and Bruce, when we would take it upon ourselves to ask at restaurants if they used peanut products. Even if I knew I couldn't understand the totality of what it meant to live with a fatal allergy, I could empathize with just wanting to be like everyone else. I reasoned that in the end, you weren't like everyone else, and that if you wanted to keep living, you'd have to just endure the constant preemptive questions and making sure. I was aware that this was logical talk about a very emotion-charged reality, and that it wasn't necessarily very helpful to you, which is perhaps why I kept it to myself. I suppose, though, that in my mind the finality of the threat you faced ended up trumping any other considerations. There didn't seem to be any "wiggle-room" with what you faced. It wasn't like a dangerous sport where talent and skill could navigate between great enjoyment and serious injury. You weren't in control of this, as much as you might want to be, and though I didn't want you to have to obsess over food or constantly confront the threat to your body, I thought that you did need to recognize that big limit. When you rejected our protectiveness, or tried to gloss over the matter, it made me nervous and irritated. I didn't know how to tell you that though I knew you wanted to be free of all the worry – yours, and the heavier kind that we laid on you – I needed you to keep giving a clear sign that you cared for your life.

Perhaps that's simple selfishness. I am sure that at times my concern was a personal comfort gained at the expense of a greater burden on you. But even if I weren't someone who takes responsibility very much to heart, I don't believe I could have acted, and been, otherwise with my little brother.

(No story from other brother)

Why Me?

I come from an island in a river of a land with hot summers and cold winters. Montreal was once a seasonal home and farm to the Mohawk people, who had and have a reputation for being among the feistier aboriginals. It received waves of French, British, African-Americans, Irish, Scottish, Chinese, Armenians, Mediterraneans, Eastern Europeans, and still more since my grandparents – of the latter two categories – boated over.

Our ancestors are famous eaters, lovers, neurotics, artists, scholars, capitalists, and humanitarians; dividers and uniters of people; carriers of a select tradition and of so many cultural influences.

For any immigrant, it can take a few generations to fit in with a land's more established peoples and build home, family, and fortune. For Sheyndle, Jakov, Ginia, and Josef (also known as Jean, Jack/Jacques, Gina, and Joe), there were some extra factors.

For one, Jewish ethnicity is bound to a religion which the Catholics and Protestants who have ruled Quebec and Canada can trace as an ancestor rebelled against. In various eras and places, Jews and Christians have had their fights, alliances, and detached coexistence. Many European Jews came to Quebec fleeing one such wave of conflict – in the form of fascism/exclusionism – yet met it here too, among other reactions. There was a boycott of "ethnic" businesses; a crackdown on communist groups, in which immigrants were prominent; and exclusion of non-Catholics from French schools, leading them to learn English and become really or symbolically allied with resented anglo power.

Then there is the matter of the Holocaust. You'd think it would dampen the immigrant's nostalgia for old country and family, given that there was no going back to them. But the community as I met it was still isolated, ready for the next eviction, dreaming of the new country (Israel, not Canada) where it would be safe and even have such power over others. Some elders went on about the past; others didn't breathe a word. The wound, it seems, has to heal before we can celebrate having made it to a place and time of peace and opportunity, with the descendants of all those other people who've survived war, epidemics, famine, serfdom, dispossession, assimilation, slavery, and more. Meanwhile people are busy surviving here, and that isn't always easy either.

I have often been overwhelmed by the problems of the past and wondered why on earth such trauma should exist, let alone be reperpetrated by people and cultures that suffered it. Depression, social trouble, and peanut allergy have told me that it is because sometimes this is what it takes to create something good and new.

Christmas, 1970. The Canadian government has invoked the War Measures Act, domestically, for the first time, in response to a murder and other gestures by radicals among the Quebec separatist movement. The cultural and political revolution that peaked a couple of years earlier in the influential US and France is here. An isolated, Church- and anglo-controlled society is diving into the modern world, with an Expo, Metro, and Olympics; rights for workers, tenants, women, gays, and the francophone majority. Dad and Mom make a baby.

They're in the process of moving from a modest Jewish neighbourhood to a rich Protestant one that's a target of political violence. They may still have some sympathies with the new Quebecois socialism, if not its ethnic nationalism. They've already rejected Zionism and scripture, Dad having grown up with the religion but not grandparents, aunts, or uncles; Mom, with a few relatives but little of the culture; both, with families that could ill afford to bicker, but did. As I grow up, being Jewish seems to have more problems than benefits. When people ask about my ethnicity, I make one up.

On the way to a radio conference in Toronto, Andrew and I get to talking about roots. His are African-Caribbean; mine are few, I say wistfully. He asks if I've tried to build any relationships with relatives. No, I haven't, I say, feeling foolish. I don't know how to begin. But he understands.

After a good night's sleep, I call Mom and ask if she can put me in touch with Grandmummy, who lives in Toronto. It's been years since we've talked. She doesn't have a good reputation in our home. "Okay." Mom says. And, after a pause: "But don't ask about my father." Jack died of a heart attack before I was born. He and Grandmummy had a stormy marriage. That's about all I know. I can't believe we have secrets just like any other family. I want to find out, and to heed Mom's wishes.

A surprisingly gracious and cheerful woman answers the door and invites me in. Much is forgiven without needing to be said. In subsequent visits, it emerges that Jacques from France was Jakov from Montreal, a businessman and artist who could be both loving and abusive. Some time after he died, Grandmummy's new love was transferred to Toronto, and she asked my folks to buy her house in that old Jewish neighbourhood. They declined. Mom was disowned. Then she got pregnant with me.

Why's Mom always stressed? I wish she'd quit smoking and eat something. Why does she do that? I need her. The food feels good but it's got something in it that feels bad. Dad's away a lot and often comes home spent. My oldest brother's mean; I wish he'd like me and am afraid of him and mad at him too. The other brother's my buddy for a long time and then suddenly he's not. The home is ours and there's always food. Mom takes care of me and Dad plays with me and sticks up for me when he can. We have hired help and few visitors. I feel loved and Mom and Dad seem to love each other too. Though they fight at the dinner table and I don't like it – or having to face my brother there every night. School's okay: I have friends and am doing well.

On to high school, some time in the first year. A lot of my old classmates are here, but they're starting to act different and their bodies are changing before mine. They have friends and fun things to do outside of school. I'm home a lot, with TV; at school, with teachers. My hero's Ken Dryden of the Montreal Canadiens: the best goalie of the best team in hockey; he's also studying law so he'll have a career when he retires, not like the others – and older folks in general – for whom they say it's all downhill after 35. I play a lot of sports too, and feel good. Some people say I'm too competitive. I like scoring and saving. I've got strong tastes and opinions too.

Mom goes back to school, to become the first woman in the family to get a PhD. She's almost done, then quits smoking. My brother and I help type and layout her thesis, using skills we learned playing at Dad's office, and sit in on her defense. She wins, 2 to 1. Her focus moves away from home. Dad's around more, and we're having good times.

We eat more "health food" than the rest of the family or most people I know. Still, it feels heavy; the city, polluted. Later we'll get more organic farms, bulk food shops, ethnic restaurants, and pollution controls, and I'll discover camping, hiking, cycling, hitchhiking, gardening, building, fix-iting, and touching. I know my way around the city but not the "nature" from which a lot of things come, and feel an unease no alarm system, medicine, or cleanser can cure.

One day at a school assembly Lucas gets his nose in front of my elbow and hemorrhages half an hour. Admin suspends me and parents send me to a psychologist. I can't be and see myself as a normal teenage male. I always seem to be thinking, apologizing, feeling crappy.

Before long I stop eating in the cafeteria with the other kids. At elementary school there was a food service – gross, but with some things I started to like, different from what I got at home, and the same as everyone else. Here we pack lunch; sometimes it's a treat but if I don't like it there's nothing else and either way people make fun of it. Same thing with my clothes. I start to hate most of the typical North American foods of the day, like macaroni and cheese, potato salad, and tuna sandwiches; limp ingredients thrown together by people who don't seem to like or know how to cook,

The Sprouted Peanut Vaccine and Other Stories

and a nagging sense that even if I deny my body's needs and act like everyone else I'll still be only superficially accepted. When teased I cry and go eat in one of the school's private bathrooms. It's the one place I know where I can lock the door and my body isn't a shame to anyone, with needs and likes that may be distinctive to me, my lineage, or my species.

I still have friends over for dinner, play, or homework, and like to see how they do things in their homes. It's good to be invited, but what if they offer something with peanuts or that I just don't like? I don't want to hurt their feelings or get sick. Sometimes I do get sick, either because they didn't understand or because I didn't ask. And when I do, I often try to hide it. When I come home, Mom asks what I ate and if I liked it. Visits become fewer and further between. I become pickier still but am not the only one and start to say so.

Mom says she likes cooking and many nights makes different things for each of us. At some point it becomes an issue how we can't keep demanding and complaining without saying thank you. I try to make it up to her, recognizing the demands of cooking, cleaning, and child-rearing when she also wants to have a career, like many women. Mom says she married Dad because he respected her. He beams. Somehow it never becomes an issue to ask him how was your day and wouldn't a shoulder-rub be nice?

Age 34

Dream. I'm back in that high school bathroom. But light is coming in, the door is open – no, it's been removed. By me.

I stop stashing sweets and stealing my brother's porno magazines to share with friends. I start sneaking out of school. Down the hill to the souvlaki parlour and the video arcade. When I come back, amazingly, teachers and admin don't crack down. Maybe because they feel for me, not just 'cause I'm a good student. Whatever I can master alone, I do: words, numbers, objects, rituals; slap shot, jump shot, slugging, volleying.

One week, we're visited by recruiters from three prestigious colleges. The vice-principal encourages me to apply. We have to write an essay. I say I want to be a Renaissance Man and major in chemistry. I'm doing well in that subject, my teacher's hip and competent, and quietly I wonder if I can cure my allergy. Princeton, New Jersey, writes back to offer me a spot; the other two decline. Who cares! I've got a ticket out of here and into being somebody. My folks are proud but think I should wait a year. My brothers don't approve so much and agree I'm too young. I want them to support me and like me.

The next year is spent in CEGEP, Quebec's pre-university college system. Nicole is my first girlfriend; a whole, beautiful adult with whom, apparently, I am one too. Having a partner lightens my mood and load. In ball hockey, there's Anand. My underdog team knocks his out and ties the stars up 2-2 in the dying moments of the championship game. Then they cheat blocking our winning goal. As coach and goalie I scream "penalty shot!" As league co-president (and chief statistician) I say "that's not in the rule book." Guess who wins.

It's not bad at all, really. Finally, I can choose my classes and teachers, and some become friends – like Ken, from West Africa. There are people who seem to be happy and love me for who I am. I'm not so sure I want to leave any more. Something's still gnawing at me. I go.

It doesn't take a week at Princeton to know it's not the place for me. I'm shy and gentle, and so are many of these folks. Across different values and ways, we connect. But a lot of us seem to be missing the same pieces.

At the end of the year I get a Summer job, with one of the government's environmental quality labs. It's my first time. The pay is good, place is pleasant, and team seems to know and like what they're doing. We get along and I keep some distance, like by skipping lunch.

Next year, similar scenario, with even stronger doubts about going back to school, and an offer to stay on with the lab. It's like my dream come true, and my nightmare: what if I try, and fail? Back to New Jersey, I say. No, back to Montreal. No, New Jersey. No, Montreal. No... I smoke my first half-pack of cigarettes, and arrive at Princeton – seven hours away – fifteen hours later. When the semester begins, I start drinking coffee. Never had that family habit, either. Take so much I practically get an ulcer. Go for tests. Nothing turns up.

In the past twenty-five months I've had two brushes with death from peanuts and one from overdrinking, plus a fire in my bedroom and time lying in the middle of the road wondering...

I crack. Cut class, play pool, make friends. We watch *The Simpsons*, listen to Nirvana, and protest the Gulf War. Sons and daughters of parents who, for all of their success, for ethnic or other reasons, haven't made it into the establishment, we're mad about the price we, they, and the planet have paid in trying to live up to that model. Now the economy's in recession, a bachelor's degree isn't worth as much as they said it would be, permanent jobs with benefits are being replaced with contracts, and loans still have to be repaid. We talk of issues more than feelings. In the ensuing years, activism and professionalism will remain my lifestyle. They may not build lasting relationships or a good nest, but they sure do burn a backlog of bile.

Upon graduation, I apply for dozens of technical jobs in Canada and Europe. It takes months to get a low-end position with a private environmental testing lab. They don't seem to care about the environment or their workers. I don't understand why I have to wait to show what I can do and am frustrated with slow, superficial change to deep, pressing human and ecological problems that it turns out have also been happening in me. Leaving my lover at 6 am to commute two hours just doesn't seem worth it. One day that I actually make it out the door on time, walk to the subway, pay my fare, and wait for the train, I stop and hear the music.

A Bulgarian flutist's playing on the other side of the turnstiles. I love world music! and have been hosting programs of it on community radio for several years now. Back out that gate I go; listen good, meet Vasil, and book an interview; then go to work and get fired before I can quit. Outside the lab, there are exciting things to share. Good thing I kept my tutoring and volunteer work. Some day Mom and Dad will understand why I keep choosing time and relationships, even when it means less money and objects, and how that can also help people. Some day I will too.

It's been one year since the day they came to my graduation, I first saw Dad walk with a cane, and he and I flew back to see the Canadiens win the last of their league-leading twenty-four championships. His quietly building arthritis had suddenly taken over; ever since, I've been reckoning with how he and I won't be young and healthy forever, at least not without study and effort. And resolving to nourish my inner child. In a way, it's what I've been doing since I turned sixteen, when I realized I'd spent the last years of my childhood trying to catch up to my brothers and schoolmates, and it's what I do every time I get very sick.

It hasn't been brought to my attention or praised so much that I am also tall, strong, handsome, sociable, smart, hard-working, light-skinned, and male. Doubt in body deepens each time Mom asks if I'm eating enough protein; Dad, if I need new shoes; or the paper, if a gene or drug can cure this disease. It eases as Mom treats most things herself, instead of going or sending us to the hospital; Dad gets bodywork and meditation instead of an operation; and together we walk and talk, edges rounding, grateful to be alive and know ourselves and each other. There is also pain, humiliation, and conflict.

Many years on, I feel I am losing the battle. Dried up, as if having used my well of sexual energy to heal the past. Time for another resolution: hand off the aboriginal-support radio show and finish the family tree. My relationships have been based on asking for and offering help, from a standpoint of trying to change. Now I want peers and living as-is. For years I've been the only son in town;

when a brother moves back, I get ready to go. "Why Africa?" some ask. "To live with people," I say.

Everywhere, a favourite topic of conversation is similarities and differences between their land and mine. It's often assumed I've had an easier life, and that's true in many respects, even given that I live modestly for a Canadian. "But often we make a lot because we spend and owe a lot and are largely to our own devices." They are shocked that successful, retirement-age people like my parents still work, by choice or necessity, and that many of their peers live alone, in seniors' homes, far from family.

When I get back, Dad says he's going for the operation, after all. I fight it, then feel it's right – for both of us. Jews, like West Africans and perhaps anyone else with an identity reinforced by survival of trauma, can be fiercely loyal to family and tribe, yet impassioned by the past to get theirs now. It's been hard for me to realize my own life matters first – to, as they say in travel, put on my oxygen mask or live vest before helping others with theirs, if needed, in an emergency.

Being in love with Belinda helps. It's a second chance to learn adult love, with the child's trust and intelligence still intact. We have many things in common and complement each other well too. It makes for a good community, which in turn keeps the relationship fresh and reveals its full meaning. One day, something goes very wrong, making love, and somehow I know what it is: abuse. Not that I've ever been a victim of it, as far as I know. Many women friends have. I start to wonder about me – and this brother, that stranger, or that family friend. At first I think there has to have been a clear physical act for it to be legitimate. Like so many of my illnesses, it was probably "just" emotional. Maybe all the harder, then, to name and cure.

I like commuting to Belinda's place across town, and how it is too when she moves three blocks away. We plan a big trip. She gets pregnant. An amazing two weeks pass. We agree on abortion but I'm surprised I'm almost ready to be a father. Later, traveling, we meet more good people and places. She goes back to her hometown and I to mine, with some other destinations along the way. We still talk about a future together, and visit, as our different directions become clear. It's a friendly separation. Maybe everyone thinks they get the tough half in these situations. I miss her and need her, and am happy for her and our friendship.

One night I head out to a poetry reading of an acquaintance who keeps inviting me to things and I feel bad because I don't go because I don't want to. A car door opens as I bike by and goes into my knee; I flip and land on my helmet. Before that it was an amazing time with my new roommate Andrea in our beautiful, warm home. Now she meets me at the hospital, with a little medicinal tea and brightness. I'm in a wheelchair, thinking "this could be my life now" and that's virtuous.

Off my feet for a few weeks, it becomes easier to ask for help. Sometimes that feels good and sometimes I wish they and their advice would go away. Enough being a victim! Hadn't I just been wanting to learn to swim, after all these years afraid of drowning and unable to share water fun? It's one thing I can do now. Andrea's there for that, and to reintroduce me to contact improvisation – a mix of modern dance, martial arts, and therapeutic touch. I always wanted to feel strong and beautiful; when I played hockey, I did. It was messy and totally in-the-moment. I just missed having someone watch me. Dance has it all.

I get better. Months later, pain returns in the leg that was hit. Nothing shows up on tests. Out dancing one night, suddenly I can't move. This will keep happening, periodically, for a couple of years. It is eerily familiar: Dad too has a twinge in the right sciatic nerve. The insurance board rejects my claim for compensation. Like it was as a kid, I need help, and despair at how someone with the authority to give it doesn't know how or refuses to because they disagree with what I feel. Yet something has changed. Family and community have taught me about many kinds of health care. Shiatsu and osteopathy are especially helpful, and filter into my whole way of living. Weird instincts awaken and work. Some pain and immobility linger. There's gotta be an emotional aspect: this knee, torn by running in opposite directions, to achieve everything and please everybody.

Damn it! Dad, Mom, I know you never asked me to take on your pains. I did it to help you, because they were bothering me. I never felt like I could do enough. Those must have been some hard times you came through. Sorry if I haven't appreciated that enough. I hope you like this story, feel good about my life, and enjoy yours.

And to whoever had that party where Ben introduced me to Hélène who'd refer me to Michelle who'd help me remember and sort a lot of this out, in five years of body-mind therapy, thank you. If I had one healing method to recommend, other than research and instinct, it would be hers. With guidance and touch, and simply by slowing down, I tune in to what is unseen or unheard in what I and we do and say, in a way that makes it easier to get along, make good choices, and see the opportunities that present themselves, even in a past I might not have chosen.

The Biology of Stress and Pleasure

At the top of the stem where brain meets spine, the hypothalamus lies in wait. For reports from detectors of the quality of temperature, hydration, nourishment, heart function, breathing, vision, and energy in the body. It can respond with instructions to keep, raise, lower, and maybe even alter one or the other, by mobilizing what is already in the body or by getting the body to ingest or excrete something. The goal is balance. In other words: the *central and peripheral nervous systems* relate with the rest of the body through *neurotransmitters* and *hormones* to achieve *homeostasis*, and the hypothalamus is the main director.[212]

Most stresses are meant to be short-lived messages to make some adjustment toward greater safety and health. When they become entrenched, for example by birth defect, injury, abuse, exhaustion, deprivation, or intensive use of potent foods, medicines, or drugs, the ability to receive sensation, accurately interpret it, effectively act on it, get feedback, and fine-tune may be impaired. From here it is a short step to hyperactivity, depression, anxiety, insomnia, oversex, undersex, obesity, anorexia, and other emotional-physical illnesses, and a contributing step to allergy, autism, diabetes, high blood pressure, asthma, chronic fatigue, fibromyalgia, and other illnesses often considered to be purely physical. By the same token, in more or less time, each of these illnesses can be traced to an imbalance which can be fixed, even if that imbalance has changed in the meantime.

The hypothalamus has also been called the pleasure centre, where you might find junkies, nymphos, or hardbodies lining up for feel-good substances it hurts to do without. Adrenaline, made from *dopamine*. Dopamine and *phenyl ethylamine*, made from *phenylalanine*. Phenylalanine, supplied by foods, particularly avocadoes, peanuts, legumes, nuts, grains, leafy vegetables, dairy, poultry, fish, and shellfish, many of which also happen to be rich in arachidonic acid and protein. Phenylalanine is also a metabolite of the artificial sweetener aspartame, and there is a debate as to whether or not aspartame can permanently damage brain chemistry. Some people *(phenylketonurics)* are totally or partly unable to metabolize phenylalanine, presumably for genetic reasons. In this way, it and/or its metabolites accumulate in blood. Many are neurotoxins. These people are more likely than average to have hyperactivity, impaired mental development, and eczema.[213] Phenylalanine imbalance, in any person, may be related to arthritis, headaches, depression, high blood pressure, Lupus, Parkinson's disease, insomnia, and learning disability.[214]

This small part of the brain is also a source of inflammatory histamine and soothing *serotonin*. Quick fixes for serotonin include sugar, starch, sex, exercise, stimulants like amphetamine and methylphenidate *(Ritalin)*, selective serotonin reuptake inhibitors like fluoxetine *(Prozac)*, and serotonin breakdown inhibitors like positive ions emitted by TV and computer screens.[215]

Going to Seed

The morphine's wearing off, and Dad's acting a little funny. He's gotta be in a lot of pain, and who knows if he'll make it over the hump. He's just had his hip replaced. The shock-absorbing cartilage on the old one was worn to the bone. In the sun room, all of the curtains are drawn and the windows are closed. I don't like it, and start going off to myself about this and that of his other penchants.

I'm sick of death and feeling unable to handle – I mean, live – life. Maybe I had to withdraw, to know myself and stop being overloaded by stimulation most people seem to find normal. Now sauce, sun, clean air, wide horizons, live music, fresh fruit, and crowds taste good, often. They take me far from home, yet feel like a homecoming. This, in retrospect, is partly what West Africa, the Mediterranean, and Latin America were about. The people from those places, as I'd met them in Canada, had seemed so healthily lively. When I got there, I felt it even more. But there was also a quiet, crushing – and familiar – despair, in this case having to do with few opportunities for advancement and much early death and suffering from hunger, disease, road accidents, and war.

I had also been attracted by the women. Then I realized I didn't know how to date! So much of what I'd learned – like, how in some circles it's cool to be a stud and in others, a feminist – seemed like posturing. At least I'd gotten the bit about having fun and protecting someone. It's just, no one had ever made clear my value and responsibility as bearer of a genetic, financial, and reputational heritage.

In Benin and Ghana we ate more or less the same starches every day; in Tunisia, Italy, and Colombia there was that plus an abundance of fresh, colourful produce. I liked both. And I was surprised how quickly people ate; often separately, in pecking order.

It did a lot to check my complaints about what's missing from life in the First World today, and to relieve expectations of what having and being and doing enough is and looks like – expectations so strong I can deny how I feel trying to live up to them and be afraid of what would probably be better.

It also gave me a taste of being regular, what with all those new critters in my gut! So long had I struggled with tension, pain, and bleeding inside, to the point of worrying about colon cancer, going for tests, and (again) finding nothing. Maybe something had been brewing on a low level. Maybe it was just stress. Feels like carrying dead weight and wanting to be rid of it before being wholly ready to. Looks like a tree cut down in its prime. My family. But the stump shoots out new growth and it's got extra room, sun, and rain to grow; the plant bolts to seed in drought season; and I get powerfully aroused when very sick with fever. The taste of death, it seems, speeds us to reproduce. They even say in French that the creation of life tends to come with a little delicious, orgasmic death (*la petite mort*).

Four
The Evolutionary Role of Allergy

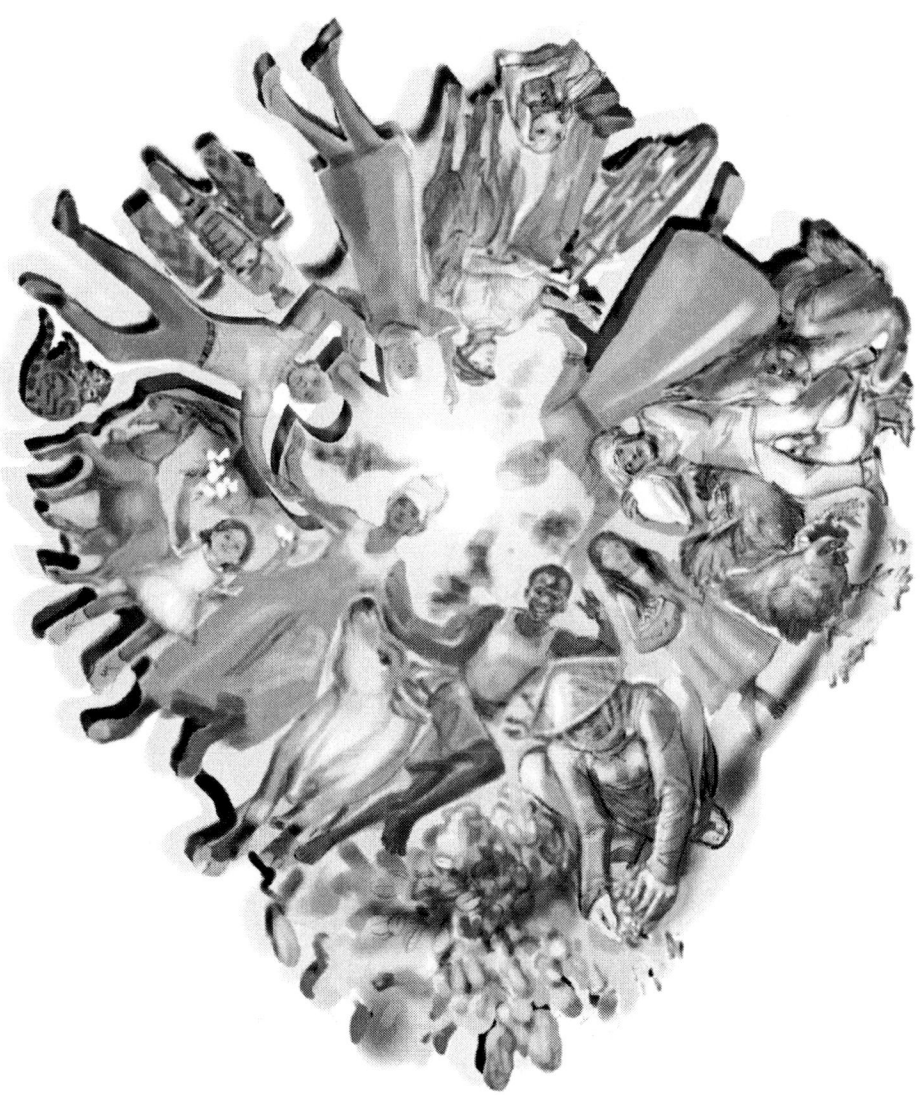

The Sprouted Peanut Vaccine and Other Stories

The Sprouted Peanut Vaccine and Other Stories

Turning the Tables

It's shiatsu school graduation. We're asked to bring something to give away, upon drawing a classmate's name from a hat. I pack up my beautiful, expensive maps of the energy channels of the body. They go to Frédérique; from Anne I get an aloe plant.

Two years on, business is still slow. People ask how it's progressing and I'm embarrassed to answer. Something our teacher Michel said or somehow communicated comes back to me: I am going to make it, because at any given moment I am an appropriate, available person for at least some other people. Because that's what I am for myself. Not necessarily "the best" or even "good." I cut down on advertising, with no loss of business. I tell people, "I like my work and it seems to be helping others." Forget all those expectations from books read or not gotten around to reading. I throw them in a box.

Years later, I want to open that box and see what it says about how I've been living.

Blood Type, Body Type, Feels Good

There are four major variations in the genes that relate to our blood: A, B, AB, and O. These have to do with the presence or absence of two markers *(antigens)*, called A and B, as can be determined by a routine clinical test.

These are antigens in the same sense as a food, microbe, or other biological substance: upon first exposure, the immune system produces antibodies to them; upon subsequent exposure, those antibodies react. Type O people have anti-A and anti-B bodies, so tend to reject A, B, or AB blood. Type As have anti-B bodies, so don't do well with B or AB blood. Bs have anti-As, so shouldn't receive A or AB. ABs have none of these antibodies, so can accept anybody's blood (as long as their Rhesus factors are also compatible). This makes ABs *universal acceptors*, with high immunity to many diseases and less incidence of autoimmune disease, including allergy; and Os, *universal donors*.[216]

The blood types developed as people were exposed to different climates, foods, and mates. Type O has been around for at least 50 000 years, since hunter-gatherer, relatively carnivorous days in Africa. Their antibodies may have developed as protection against the wide range of animal-borne parasites thus encountered. Type A appeared in near and central Asia 25 000 years ago, as agrarian, densely populated, relatively omnivorous living appeared. Type B arose in central Asia, about 15 000 years old, and AB is barely 1000.[217] As a result, ethnic groups today have different proportions of the four types, and each type remains built for a certain diet, lifestyle, and environment.[218] Genes for blood type and food metabolism remain close neighbours on chromosome pair #9 of the 23 found in most cells of the body.[219]

In Ayurveda, people are considered to be some combination of the vata, pitta, and kapha archetypes. As discussed earlier, this is figured out by looking at various physical and emotional qualities, from body shape to system functioning, temperament, and lifestyle.[220] Certain foods can be recommended to correct imbalances or maintain balance, because each food's energy is likewise understood as being relatively vata, pitta, and/or kapha. Over the long term, then, people can make choices that affect the nature of their bodies and feelings, as they cycle or evolve with the seasons, aging, and other processes.

According to these systems, I have blood type A and am relatively vata/pitta in nature.

Out of all the foods you or I may have access to nowadays, I'm going to see how those that make me feel best and worst – not necessarily that I like or dislike for taste, appearance, or texture – fit the blood and body type recommendations.

	Recommended for blood type A?[221]	Recommended for body type vata / pitta?[222]	Feels good last 24 months?
Whole grains	Some	Some / Most	Most
Amaranth	Yes	-	Yes
Buckwheat	Yes / Neutral	No	No
Oats	Neutral	Yes	Yes
Quinoa	Neutral	Yes	Yes
Grain products	Some	Some / Most	Some
Popcorn	No / Neutral	No	Yes
Wheat bread	No / Neutral	Yes	No
Legumes	Some	Few / Most	Few
Mung beans	Neutral	Yes	Yes
Meat	None	Most / Few	Most
Bison	No	Yes / No	Yes
Lamb	No / Neutral	Yes / No	Yes
Pork	No	Yes / No	No
Dairy	Few	Most / Some	Few
Cow	No	Yes	No
Eggs	None	Most / Some	Few
Fish	Some	Most / Few	Most
Haddock	No / Neutral	Yes / No	Yes
Herring	No / Neutral	Yes / No	Yes
Mackerel	Yes	Yes / No	Yes
Shellfish	None	Most / Few	Some

The Sprouted Peanut Vaccine and Other Stories

	Recommended for blood type A?[221]	Recommended for body type vata / pitta?[222]	Feels good last 24 months?
Root vegetables	Some	Most / Few	Most
Beet	Neutral	Yes / No	Yes
Potato	No	No / Yes	Yes
Turnip	Yes	Yes / No	Yes
Bulb vegetables	Most	Most / Few	Some
Onion	Yes	Yes / No	Yes
Fruit vegetables	Few	Few / Some	Some
Eggplant	No / Neutral	No / Yes	Yes
Leaf vegetables	Most	Some / Few	Most
Endive	Neutral	-	Yes
Lettuce	Yes / Neutral	No / Yes	Yes
Spinach	Yes	No	Yes
Fruit	Some	Most / Some	Some
Avocado	Neutral	Yes / No	Yes
Grape	Neutral	Yes	No
Lemon	Yes	Yes / No	Yes
Plum	Yes	Yes	No
Nuts	Some	Most / None	Some
Nut products	Some	Most / Few	Few
Seeds	None	Most / Few	Few
Seed products	None	Most / Few	Few
Sesame butter	Neutral	Yes / No	No
Oils	Some	Most / Some	Some
Flax	Yes	Yes / No	Yes
Olive	Yes	Yes / No	Yes
Sesame	Yes / Neutral	Yes / No	No
Herbs	None	Most / Some	Most
Basil	Neutral	Yes / No	Yes
Bay leaf	Neutral	Yes / No	Yes
Marjoram	Neutral	-	Yes
Saffron	Neutral	Yes	Yes

	Recommended for blood type A?[221]	Recommended for body type vata / pitta?[222]	Feels good last 24 months?
Spices	Few	Most / Some	Most
Anise	Neutral	-	Yes
Caraway	Neutral	-	Yes
Cayenne	No / Neutral	Yes / No	Yes
Cloves	Neutral	Yes	Yes
Ginger	Yes	Yes / No	Yes
Condiments	Some	Some	Some
Grey sea salt	Neutral	Yes / No	Yes
Honey	Neutral	Yes	Yes
White salt	Neutral	-	No
White or brown sugar	No / Neutral	No	No
Drinks	Some	Some	Few
Alcohol	No / Neutral / Yes	Yes / No	No
Coffee	Yes	- / No	No
Fruit juice	No / Neutral / Yes	Yes	No

The Ayurvedic prescription seems to have more fits than misfits, while the blood type one has equal amounts of both. I'm not saying if they – or my experience – are valid or not. All are here for a reason, with subtleties such a chart can't convey. Probably, any system that takes a rich and diverse view of our bodies and feelings, in relationship with others' and the natural world, can work or not work for us, for however long; we can keep or outgrow some of its rules, while staying true to ourselves and even to it.

Horny Like the Bull

There's an expression in English, "to take the bull by the horns." It means, to confront a seemingly impossible or dangerous challenge, head-on.

That's what I've been doing, in many respects, all my life: forcing myself to grow, in the rush to feel better; sensing people around me live so fast and intense, and not wishing to see myself as falling into the same trap; yet often finding another way to do it, like making activism my business or foods my pills.

Not that it's bad to take bulls by horns sometimes. It can be a neat way to learn limits and feel alive. But it can be tiring and frustrating too. I couldn't solve peanut allergy alone, and the cures felt as lonely as the disease.

You know that book about tapping into your inner power, *Women Who Run with the Wolves* (by Claudia Pinkola-Estes)? Well, I don't feel quite like I'm running with my bull; more, that I am the bull.

Animals and I get along pretty good. For years I'd go do some farmwork or shepherding, usually in the Summer, and one place I went back to was Audrey's up in the Canadian Shield. She and Joel had left good jobs in the city to raise sheep on the rock, and – as it turned out – let Joel get sick and then better. He wasn't given much chance of surviving colon cancer, but a diet of raw organic foods and coffee enemas was helping. They called it the Gerson plan, and shared some of the foods, like mango-gingko-wheat-grass juice that made me and my pee positively glow.

Now there's a word and an experience of which I've been as terrified as "peanut." Merely seeing "cancer" in an ad or headline has made me shudder, look away, and pray it won't get me. Yet somehow now it feels fine to add that book to my box.

Cancer

Most living creatures, ourselves included, are made of cells, some generic and some specialized. These have various ways and rates of copying their flesh and instructions for the next generation. Many cancers involve copying errors made going too fast. One of the big questions in trying to cure and prevent them is, how do good instructions go bad? There is the idea of carcinogenic substances, like free radicals, that have the ability to alter DNA (*deoxyribonucleic acid*), and of substances, like anti-oxidants, that can prevent if not repair damage.

Max Gerson was a German doctor who developed successful dietary treatments for tuberculosis, lupus, cancer, and other diseases in the first half of the twentieth century. He was also one of a crew of First-Worlders (with Albert Schweitzer, Robert McCarrison, Roger Williams, and Weston Price, soon to be discussed) to note the sudden appearance or rise of these and other diseases as people switched from whole and/or traditional foods and activities to refined and/or novel ones.

According to his theory, cancer comes from a progressive poisoning of the liver, impairment of the intestines, and weakening of the body; not from a missing essential substance (like a vitamin, enzyme, or hormone) or toxic foreign one. When a critical level of poisoning is reached, an allergic reaction kicks in. At that moment, enzymatic activity is at a low. Though bad symptoms appear, it is actually the beginning of a healing cleanse.[223]

Gerson's diet is meant to help the process along. Foods are taken in ways that preserve their life energy and nutrient balance; enemas may also be given. In this way, enzymes reactivate, the liver regenerates, histamine released into circulation as tumours dissolve gets neutralized or eliminated, and further poisoning is avoided. Three-quarters of the food consists of:

☆ Fruit: raw, dried, or lightly cooked, not frozen, canned, or sulfured;

- ☆ Vegetables: raw, dried, or stewed in their own juices, not fried, pressure-cooked, frozen, canned, smoked, or sulfured;
- ☆ Whole grains;
- ☆ Natural sweeteners: in moderation.

Originally, calf's liver juice was also a key component. However, raw animal products can have some particular microbes and parasites; an outbreak of *campylobacter* led the Gerson Institute to drop this item from the diet.

If health improves, additional foods can be introduced in moderation:

- ☆ Dairy, though not cream or salted or spiced cheese;
- ☆ Meat and fish, though not canned, smoked, or salted;
- ☆ Eggs;
- ☆ Nuts;
- ☆ Herbs.

Stimulants and poisons are forbidden throughout:

- ☆ Nicotine;
- ☆ Most alcohols;
- ☆ Coffee;
- ☆ Most teas;
- ☆ Most spices;
- ☆ Baking soda;
- ☆ Refined salt;
- ☆ All vitamin pills except B_3 and C;
- ☆ Aluminum, from cookware.

The issue with refined salt is that it is all sodium chloride, without the other minerals found in natural salt and needed for a balanced effect in the body.[224] It's not clear where legumes fit in, except that soy is discouraged, at least in the first few months.

Gerson also used this approach for asthma, osteoarthritis, morning sickness, and some heart, spinal cord, and mental troubles.

Another school of whole-food thought applied to cancer is the *macrobiotic* one. The word means "big life" or "long life" and has been around for at least two hundred years. The practice is much older, and enjoyed a revival in early-1900s Japan; from there, it spread to the US and Europe, by way of people like George Ohsawa and Michio Kushi.

In his book on cancer prevention, Kushi echoes Gerson's understanding and finds that most of the foods good for treating the disease help avoid it in the first place. He points out that cancer is a relatively recent epidemic, even in the First World, though that may have to do with living longer as well as with changing food and lifestyle. He situates refined food within a larger problem of hypernutrition, involving too much dietary carb, protein, and fat. And he raises the issue of people consuming foods foreign to their cultures and climates. Specifically, those living in temperate zones like Japan or the US are advised to skip foods grown in or derived from the tropics and subtropics.[225]

The foods recommended for everybody are:
- ☆ Lots of grains: mostly whole and cooked as porridge; some processed (like flour and flakes); none highly refined (like white flour);
- ☆ Lots of vegetables: steamed, boiled, pressure-cooked, sautéed or baked; lots of roots, with their leafy tops; lots in the cabbage family; some in the onion family; little in the mushroom family; none in the nightshade family;[226]
- ☆ Moderate legumes: especially adzuki, chickpea, lentil, and fermented soy;
- ☆ Moderate seaweed;
- ☆ Moderate oil: mostly sesame, corn, and mustard; none highly refined;
- ☆ Moderate salt: none highly refined.

People already in good health can add:
- ☆ Moderate fish and shellfish;
- ☆ Moderate fruit, but no juice;
- ☆ Tea, but only from twigs or roasted grains;

☆ Alcohol, but only from traditional fermentation processes.

Stimulants are discouraged:
☆ Coffee;
☆ Black and herbal teas;
☆ Refined alcohols.

As an alternative to the idea of carcinogens, Kushi talks about how substances can aggravate or improve a condition of extreme yang or ying. For example, rubbing a rabbit on the ear with coal tar every day for months can make a tumour, not by damaging cells directly but because its yang nature causes the blood to send in ying antidotes whose expansive nature (as opposed to the constrictive, yang tar) makes the growth. He classifies foods as follows:

☆ Yang: most animal products, but not most dairy (only cheese); refined salt.
☆ Ying: all other dairy; fruit; refined grains; oils; spices; stimulants; sweeteners; alcohol; chemical additives; agricultural chemicals; recreational drugs; pharmaceuticals.
☆ Balanced: unrefined grains; seeds; nuts; legumes; vegetables; seaweeds; unrefined salt.

For the last couple of years, my typical breakfast has been oatmeal with spices, plus olive oil or coconut milk and maybe some honey or fruit; a typical dinner, salad plus vegetable stew with olive oil, salt, herbs, and maybe some fish, legumes, or meat; sometimes with a snack in between, of dried fruit, nuts, tea, or pop.

It seems I've gravitated toward a mostly macrobiotic and "healthy" diet. But, gee, maybe that's because I had or have cancer or some other terrible disease! You never know... but you can always worry, or not.

Wild Speculation

Bland and Lively

Seriously, now, how can someone active live on little protein and many hours between meals?

It's precisely because I felt fragile and confused – hypoglycemic, or at least afraid of lacking lasting food-energy – that I began testing my limits and what I'd heard about human nature; it's because I kept feeling better that I continued.

After all that agonizing and experimenting, it seems that much of my appetite, digestion, elimination, energy level, sleep quality, immunity, and feelings has nothing to do with what I eat or whatever else I do to try to heal. Each has ups and downs owing to my nature, the weather, daily experiences, or things that remain a mystery. And each has a stable baseline, which good, simple habits help me tune into and keep.

I needed a lot of sugar and spice to keep up with a frenetic world, until I no longer could. Secure in the knowledge that they are there if wanted, I can choose to do without, and discover that they are already in me. Taking in less, but still enough, for the first time I feel full.

Unwittingly, my search for simplicity has also been about grounding anxiety: from early awareness of my mortality, to a family climate of vulnerability, rapidly changing and uneven social fabric, and job serving people in high-pressure career tracks.

Allergic and Not

Sometimes I have wondered if my illness were a punishment from God or Science for having done something wrong; other times I've held it high like a trophy, as proof I'm innocent of whatever bore me this way. When not wanting to share a meal or build a relationship, I have heard myself say, "watch out, because a drop of peanut can send me to the hospital and it'll be your fault;" when wanting to share or relate, "I have a problem with peanuts but it's getting better;" when unsure, "I can handle it," or no mention of allergy at all.

Before setting out to bike across America, I also told people different stories, and they reacted in a likewise wide array of ways, from "don't do it, you fool!" to "go, you daredevil!" It just came out that way, alternately defying and encouraging expectations with which I was uncomfortable.

Recently, on the way to poor and reputedly dangerous places far away, better words came: "I feel this is right for me, and I care about how you feel.

"I don't seek extreme risk.

"I seek to confirm my feeling that some apparently extreme risks can be safely taken, with lasting benefits, such as new confidence or ideas.

"I seek to confirm my feeling that many of us downplay the risks of 'civilized' life, like crossing traffic or steeping in loneliness.

"I seek to confirm my feeling that trying to live with no risk – indeed, in denial of the risks – is very dangerous. As when eating to the point of obesity or becoming so rich as to constantly fear theft.

"I seek to live with the moderate risks that people have always evolved with and the particular, low-level risks of today.

"In this way, I will be more at peace most of the time and better able to respond to true danger."

My allergy might put it this way: "I don't seek pointless adrenaline-rushes; I'm trying to learn how to stop hepping up on adrenaline; I'm already high as it is; this is partly for lack of legitimate outlets; it's healthy for me to relax; I'll function better in routine and extreme situations alike."

Conscious and Unconscious

My aversion to drugs has partly to do with wanting to be fully present during allergic reactions and other situations requiring my attention.

I first took diphenhydramine and epinephrine years before consciously experimenting with allergy, so don't remember their original emotional associations and tend to see them more for their physical effects. I'm confident in diphenhydramine and willing to put up with its side effects, but try to avoid epinephrine, for reasons discussed earlier.

Reading and hearsay led me to natural medicines. I wanted something that could ease reaction while letting me learn to metabolize the allergen and avoid unpleasant effects of drugs.

Calming myself is a hunch. I want a tool that works when no medicine is available and a new look at the assumption that my body can't deal alone with the allergen, at least some of the time. These tools and this process also make it easier to see emotional overload coming and nip it in the bud, or get over it when it comes.

With so many people experiencing burn-out, bad break-ups, eating disorders, and so on, I wonder how fast the cutting out has to be, or how low the threshold, before we call it "allergy" or "autism."

From what I understand of physio-psychotherapy, one thing that can make someone repeatedly misperceive signals is trauma. Because trauma, itself, can come from experiencing powerful, contradictory signals, whether in one big incident, a pattern of incidents, or a barely perceptible climate; abuse from a loved one, smiles over gritted teeth, or imperatives to "hurry up and do it perfectly."

The split tends to be between a conscious, verbalized, external message and an unconscious, felt, internal one. The latter is generally truer, and it seems to me children, animals, and wise adults are more likely to trust it. However, there can be social pressure to heed the former. Depending on how strong that is and how long it lasts or is repeated, conflict with oneself can follow.

This kind of trauma can be improved or cured by experiencing communication in which the conscious and unconscious are in harmony, often enough to get used to it as normal. That can be done from the outside in, for example with massage on skin through to muscle, fluid, and bone, and from the inside out, for example by working through the feelings that come with a given condition well enough to change how one lives it out in the world.

Because my allergy has been around for a long time and sometimes been severe, it has taken a lot of work to heal. One of my teachers said it takes a month of shiatsu to heal a year of illness. Sometimes, especially after breakthroughs, I need to rest a lot. Consciously, I relearn the trust, in body and feelings, with which it is normal to be born but which can flake off or erode at various points before or after, often unawares. My filters were clogged and junk got in my system; now I feel cleaner and am realizing I may not always have to work so hard to maintain it.

In this quiet space, inspiration comes easier – like "maybe when I got sick and blamed coconut it was really something else," "I don't feel allergic to legumes any more," or "it's okay to try a little sprouted peanut" – and I can try, deal with the consequences, and move on.

Anxious and Secure

Mom zestily retells the story of my first big peanut reaction and spends her days helping people in extreme need. It and our heritage sure made an impression on me, and I like helping people too. Both of us handle emergencies well. Maybe because they're comforting: low-level, chronic anxiety takes the form of a solvable problem, or at least one we don't have to live with full-time. And maybe too because playing offense feels different from defense.

In a home full of unnamed worries and stresses, my allergy was an epitome of constant, absolute risk. It gave the promise of a safe resting place, somewhere beyond. But it required that I, or we, never actually be able to get there. Even if the original risk may at some point have eased, fear had become a comfortable reference point I or we didn't have the confidence to leave for an unknown beyond, even if that was freedom. Fear had become the safe harbour.

Yet the framework, "peanut allergy is caused by protein, any dose can be fatal, and avoidance is the only answer," disquieted me more than it reassured; in a child-proofed playground I could still get hurt or lonely. Because I was, after all, a child. The kind who didn't like to laugh at others, because he never knew when he'd go from being "in" to being "out," or "gifted" to "hypersensitive." As to later aboriginal ("noble savage") and afro ("sexy sambo") friends, it all felt like somebody else's game of disconnection. Maybe other homes had their absolutes, like "Germans are the cause, Arabs the threat, and an exclusive Israel the answer," "Jews, Israel, and overthrow," or "Anglos, English, and an independent Quebec." Maybe I had harsh judgments that just stayed inside.

Sick and Healthy

Another of Mom's favourite stories is about how her family ate a pound of butter a week and most of her dad's family died of heart disease.

At least since I've been around, she's had trouble digesting fat, and the explanation's been that pregnancy hormones disrupted her gallbladder. But all mothers go through those changes – so there must have been some vulnerability to start with. Maybe her seemingly distinct symptoms of intolerance to animal fat and allergy to scallops both came to say, "enough of this rich food (and emotional drama), or else heart disease is coming!" And maybe my allergy is an extension of this evolutionary attempt at a safety valve.[227] For whatever reason, we both find the liver/gallbladder cleanser milk thistle helps our conditions.

Clean and Dirty

Heart disease, cancer, and some other diseases are so pervasive they might seem natural facts of life. Each kills millions of people worldwide, but there are some important socio-geographic differences:[228]

% of fatalities in high income countries	% of fatalities in mid income countries	% of fatalities in low income countries
Coronary heart disease and stroke: 26.9	Coronary heart disease and stroke: 30.6	Coronary heart disease and stroke: 16.8
Cancer of the trachea, bronchi, lung, colon, rectum, stomach, or breast: 12.8	Respiratory obstruction and lower tract infection: 10.9	Respiratory obstruction and lower tract infection: 13.1
Respiratory obstruction and lower tract infection: 8.2	Cancer of the trachea, bronchi, lung, or stomach: 5.5	HIV/AIDS: 7.5
Alzheimer and dementias: 2.7	HIV/AIDS: 3.0	Fetal and infancy problems: 6.4
Diabetes: 2.7	Fetal and infancy problems: 2.9	Diarrheal diseases: 5.4
	Road accidents: 2.6	Malaria: 4.4
		Tuberculosis: 3.8

In the sense that our bodies do these things in response to what is going on inside and outside, they are natural.

Now let's see how the people and diseases of one country can evolve:[229]

Incidence of fatalities in the US today	Incidence of fatalities in the US a century ago
Heart disease: 1 in 400 people	Pneumonia and flu: 1 in 500 people
Cancer: 1 in 500	Tuberculosis: 1 in 500
Stroke and cerebro-vascular diseases: 1 in 1700	Diarrheal diseases: 1 in 700
Respiratory obstruction: 1 in 2000	Heart disease: 1 in 700
Accidents and "adverse effects:" 1 in 3000	Stroke and cerebro-vascular diseases: 1 in 900

The Sprouted Peanut Vaccine and Other Stories

Incidence of fatalities in the US today	Incidence of fatalities in the US a century ago
Pneumonia and flu: 1 in 3000	Kidney diseases other than cancer: 1 in 1100
Diabetes: 1 in 4000	Accidents: 1 in 1400
Suicide: 1 in 9000	Cancer: 1 in 1600
Kidney diseases other than cancer: 1 in 10 000	Senility: 1 in 2000
Liver diseases other than cancer: 1 in 11 000	Diphtheria: 1 in 2000

It's hard to know how many more people have these diseases but die of something else first. In some or all cases, data may not exist.[230]

It's also a challenge to date or quantify lifestyle changes and then relate them to diseases. However, we can get an idea from technologies and theories that make new things possible.

For example, it was only in the latter 1800s and early 1900s that white bread as we know it became widespread: steel-roller milling allowed wheat's starch to be separated from its germ and bran; Louis Pasteur's biology of yeast led to commercial varieties that could replace artisanal ones or sourdough; communal bread ovens spread; transportation and communications facilitated national and international manufacturing and distribution; these could link with professional associations, government, and media to influence masses of consumers; and enough people could afford to eat the newly available or recommended foods.[231]

Among other virtues, white flour, sugar, salt, and other products looked clean, made new treats possible, and lasted forever on the shelf. Their nutritional value was debated using new theories of vitamins, minerals, carbohydrates, proteins, fats, and enzymes. It took time to track the downsides, especially when foods were introduced gradually, among an ethnically diverse population.

In the early-1900s US, for example, dentist Weston Price noticed that people seemed to be getting a lot more cavities than they used to. To find out why, he went traveling, in four continents, among tribes that had only recently begun using some of these foods. He found not only rampant tooth decay but also diabetes, tuberculosis, birth defects, mental retardation, and other diseases previously scarce or unknown. The issue wasn't necessarily that the new foods were bad, but that they were being used to excess because the alternatives were being eliminated: breastmilk, by formula; porridge, by bread; and so on.[232]

People need food that's easy to digest, but not so easy that the energy doesn't last or complementary nutrients are missing; and, among other things, we need food that stores well. Looking at cereals, and overlooking some of their differences (for example, that quinoa seeds are easier to digest than wheat but give a less versatile flour):

Form of grain	Ease of digestion	How long energy lasts	Nutritional completeness	Resistance to spoilage
White flour	High	Short	Low	High (dead)
Whole flour	Medium-high	Short-medium	Medium	Low (fully exposed)
Rolled or cut seed	Medium	Medium	High	Medium (part exposed)
Seed	Medium-low	Long	High	High (dormant)

Just as it takes time for people to accept that white flour is better than brown, it takes time to reverse opinion. Only in the 1990s, for example, did the US Food and Drug Administration overhaul its early-1900s nutrition standard of meat, dairy/eggs, carbs, and fruit/vegetables. And to this day the idea persists that, regardless of ethnicity, body type, or lifestyle, everyone needs a lot of animal protein or carefully combined plant protein.[233]

High and Low

I was drawn to carbs to feel better about an emotional and maybe physical ill, but they made me feel worse. Something similar seemed to be happening with aboriginal friends whose elders could still remember a time without sugar, flour, or alcohol; reservations, residential schools, and blood-quantum rules; substance abuse, obesity, or diabetes. And I got the feeling that the Euro-American settlers, whom it was fashionable to blame for all of this human and environmental devastation, had come here and acted this way because they too had been abused and deprived; that all of us, with excessive habits today, try to live down the past.

If we were cans of pop dropped or shaken up, we'd be ready to explode. But we're organisms; to being stuffed, blocked, and stressed, we can try to adapt. We might be able to do so in our own bodies, or we might need generations to complete the process.

Ever Changing

Some stresses and mutations help a species evolve. Like lactose tolerance: kids need calcium to grow bones and other tissues and systems, and milk is a rich source; for adult maintenance, plant sources can usually suffice. So, people of many ethnicities are born able to digest milk sugar (lactose) but lose the ability on the way to adulthood. Northern Europeans don't, and one of the explanations is that their climate prevents year-round access to good plant sources of calcium.[234]

Other mutations appear and disappear without a trace. Still others, like cancer, take on a damaging life of their own.

A few decades before Price, Russian geneticist Nikolai Vavilov and his team traveled the world to understand how our food-societies came to be. They identified eight relatively small areas, in China, India, Central Asia, the Middle East, the Mediterranean, East Africa, Central America, and northwest South America, as centres of biodiversity: almost all, temperate mountains, where extreme ranges of temperature, moisture, light, and soil provoke plenty of mutations and give mutants a choice of conditions in which best to survive.[235]

To a large extent, these coincide with the areas where we started taming plants and animals, ten to twenty thousand years ago. Agriculture made it easier to accumulate surplus, settle down, and develop other conditions of city culture *(civilization)*. All that captive energy, often unequally distributed, then spurred further developments.

Those first farmer-hunter-gatherers must have depended on their knowledge of wild creatures, just as creatures depend on theirs of us and others: plants of a species ripen at different speeds, scatter their tubers and seeds, endow them with spikes or poisons, and do other things to ensure that no predator or freak of weather can claim them all; animals have their own promiscuity, variable development, venoms, and weapons, plus the ability to run, fly, or swim, often from birth or soon after. Since then we have progressed largely by undoing those survival mechanisms. Our potatoes cluster together and chickens come home to roost; tomatoes need tutors and sheep need guard dogs. Could this have affected our own resistance to attack, famine, and disease?

Strong and Weak

In every moment, parts of us are building up and parts are breaking down. The balance changes from day to night, season to season, and birth to death. This is true of every other animal and every plant, including those that feed us. All of our rhythms, and all of theirs, are superimposed and somehow seek balance.

Biological science calls plants *producers* of matter and animals *reducers*. Each takes things apart and reassembles them to meet its needs, and the way they do this is often complementary. For example, plants consume carbon dioxide and nitrogenous waste *(humus)* to make carbs and oxygen, which animals consume to make carbon dioxide and humus.

Sugars, starches, and other carbohydrates are made from carbon, hydrogen, and oxygen. Proteins have all of these plus nitrogen and sometimes sulfur too. Relatively speaking, then, proteinaceous foods are rich in nitrogen and carbs are rich in carbon. A balance of the two is needed for plant and animal matter to grow and decay properly. Our energy, structure, hormones, and other vital features also require fat, plus enzymes that make body processes happen in a reasonable amount of time.

When I eat a lot of protein, I get more aches and pains than usual, for a day or two. It feels like the protein is revealing something that was already there, unnoticed. I feel powerful and, under that, disturbingly vulnerable; crave more protein and worry I'll lack energy; and also crave carbs, in a different way from when eating sugar or bread and craving more of the same. The best thing to do in these situations is to eat light and carby and work out. It can take four or five days to feel I've extracted all the good stuff and cleared all the waste. If I pile on more rich food before that, I can feel angrily bursting with energy and want to bolt; and, at the same time, clogged and sleepy, unable or unwanting to flee. It's like the beginning of the too-much-too-fast-too-contradictory feeling of allergy, autism, hyperactivity, and depression.

In a similar way, when I eat a lot of carbs, I often crave more of the same, whereas complex, proteinaceous food satisfies the craving. Eating too much easy carb feels like running my engine too hot, risking blow-out; adding complex fuel, like slowing and cooling it down, so the energy lasts longer.

Hmm. So digesting rich food takes a lot of energy, which light food can supply. Eventually, it gives back a lot of energy; in the meantime, something else fills the gap. So I am built to last, after all! And food can be about pleasure and security, at least as much as about anxiety – both the millennial kind and the kind that may be particular to living in the First World today.[236]

The Sprouted Peanut Vaccine and Other Stories

Hungry and Satisfied

Some alternative medics consider craving to be a symptom of allergy.[237]

How can I like a food and be unsatisfied by it? First explanation: I like stuffing my face. Second: the food is incomplete for humans. Third: it's complete, but some people don't know how to digest it fully; either they were born that way or they unlearned the ability, gradually or suddenly; so maybe they can learn or relearn it, for example by trying a new cooking method or attitude.

That falafel I couldn't get enough of came from fava beans and chickpeas. It turns out that some people are born deficient in the glucose-6-phosphate dehydrogenase (*G6PD*) enzyme needed to digest a component of favas. One of G6PD's other roles is to maintain red blood cells. If a G6PD-deficient person eats fava beans, red blood cells can suddenly die en masse, leading to anemia and/or jaundice. The disease, called *favism*, is most common among Mediterranean, African, and Southeast Asian peoples.[238]

My G6PD status hasn't been diagnosed, but I do have Gilbert's syndrome, a benign glitch in red blood cell recycling. People with Gilbert's are deficient in the liver enzyme that clears the body of bilirubin, a pigment derived from the iron-protein *(hemoglobin)* complex that, when the cells are alive and well, attracts oxygen from the lungs and delivers it throughout the body. Gilbert's syndrome has some of the same symptoms as favism, like jaundice and dark urine, and there may be a mechanistic connection.[239] People with Gilbert's syndrome are also prone to gallstones.[240] So maybe my allergy also has this to do with Mom's wonky gall bladder and my attraction to enzyme-rich foods.

Many of my cravings are nostalgic, in the sense that they are thoughts or feelings related to some memory, not to what I actually want now. I realize it the moment I go eat the food and don't feel good. The same thing applies to cravings for people, music, bike trips, and so on.

I grew up feeling hungry amid much apparent food. Later, I pursued "community," and found it feasting and laughing together. It was so good I wanted more as it went by. When I was alone or we were just hanging out quietly, I missed it and wondered where the magic had gone. It wasn't that my body wanted more; I wanted the promise of more. Hunger was comfortably familiar, like a food – that, magically, I could eat without end.

If I've tended to ditch drugs and junk food, it's not only for wanting to feel well. Because of the way I was made, I've had other ways of facing death and feeling high on life, while fearing no life-energy to spare. So I've missed out on some of the hallmark experiences of youth here today. Or maybe we're not so different, from each other and those elsewhere or before us.

Fed-up and Thrilled

From a small town in Ghana I arrive in the capital of Tunisia. First impression: wow, disposable income. Not a lot, like back home, but enough for a night out with coffee, amazing pastries, cigarettes, and no work. Why aren't they celebrating and nurturing their relative freedom and security? It's been months since I've breathed any cigarette smoke and now my lungs are full and heart is racing and I'm having too much fun to quit.

We're at one of those chic cafés, under one of those palm trees, that line the boulevard. He's smoking, like every guy here seems to, and I'm asking why. "We're pissed off," he says. Here we are, supposed to be gaining wealth and prestige from development, yet not really having many more opportunities for work, travel, and the fulfilment of other desires, and to do it we've been sacrificing our connection to land and family.

Here we are with the power to bring death near, to remember joy. Driven to achieve higher and faster, we can revolt by diminishing our capacities and celebrating our incompleteness. And so, perhaps, can those on whom we rely: crops mass-grown, alone, in orderly fashion, in water or depleted soil, pushed by fertilizer, supported by killing plants and bugs around them, cut down before their reproductive prime, shipped off, cut into parts sent in further directions, preserved before being allowed to decay, and dressed up with colours, flavours, and textures; livestock caged or fenced in tight, quick-fattened on grain, animal byproduct, and growth hormone, defended with antibiotics, disproportionately killed before their first birthday or for being male, females bred to bear twins or triplets over and over, dissected, objectified, prolonged in living death.[241]

On that farm up in the Canadian Shield, Audrey warns me not to let the sheep get at the bag of corn. "Why," I ask, eager to learn and fond of the stuff. "Because they'll gorge and get sick."[242] She also tells of factory ewes keeling over at 3 or 4 from multiplet breeding. Some of hers are over 10 years old – "and kinda friends," she says.

Grains and legumes are energy-packed compared to grasses and other plant parts on which many farm animals and their ancestors have traditionally relied. The varieties we eat may be even more manipulated than those we give to livestock. Their processed products, like meal, starch, and syrup, get into so many packaged and prepared foods, as do milk's. Allergy and intolerance spread.[243]

For aboriginals and others, Carl Barnes comes on the radio show to explain, traditional varieties have a cultural, agricultural, and nutritional value. Their starchy, fibrous nature makes them hardier crops and healthier foods than contemporary sweet corn. Their replacement coincided with the appearance of diabetes, and their reintroduction, even alongside sweet corn, helps cure and prevent it.[244]

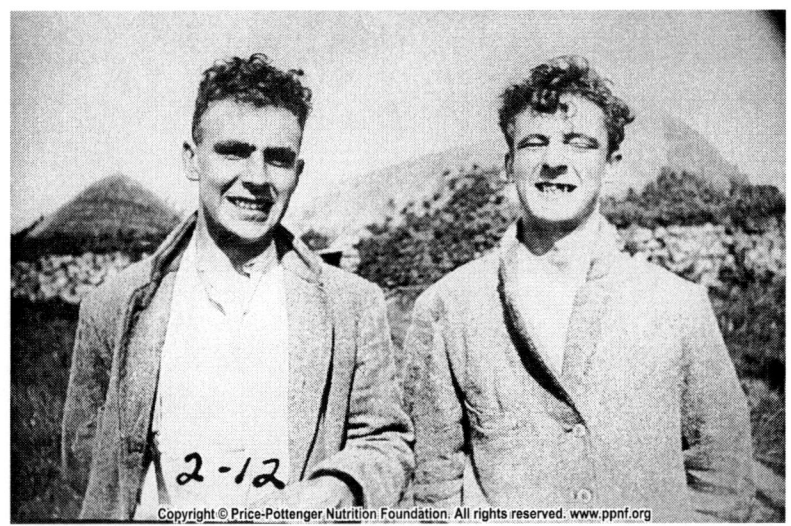

"This shows two boys; the older at the left has excellent teeth. He lived on the native diet of oat products and sea foods. His brother at the right used the imported white flour bread, sugar, jams and coffee shipped from the port about sixty miles away. These boys are on the isle of Harris.

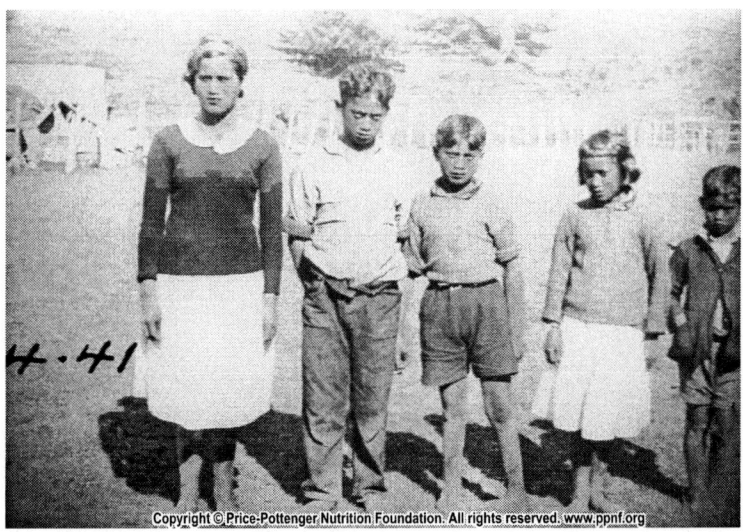

"This illustrates another important phase of this problem. Not only do errors in physical development occur in the head, but often in other parts of the body. The oldest girl to the left has a splendidly developed face and has normal feet. The second child has a marked lack of development of the middle third of the face. He has flat feet. The third child has a marked underdevelopment of the middle third of the face and he has club feet." – Weston Price

Reforming Animal Nature

In the late 1900s, American biologist Jared Diamond traveled the world asking farm animals what their recipe was for domestic success after so many years in the wild. They said,
- ☆ "Don't be fussy about food,
- ☆ "Grow up fast,
- ☆ "Mate where you live,
- ☆ "Be pleasant,
- ☆ "Don't try to escape, and
- ☆ "Accept a sociopolitical hierarchy."[245]

Five
After the Storm, Fertile Calm

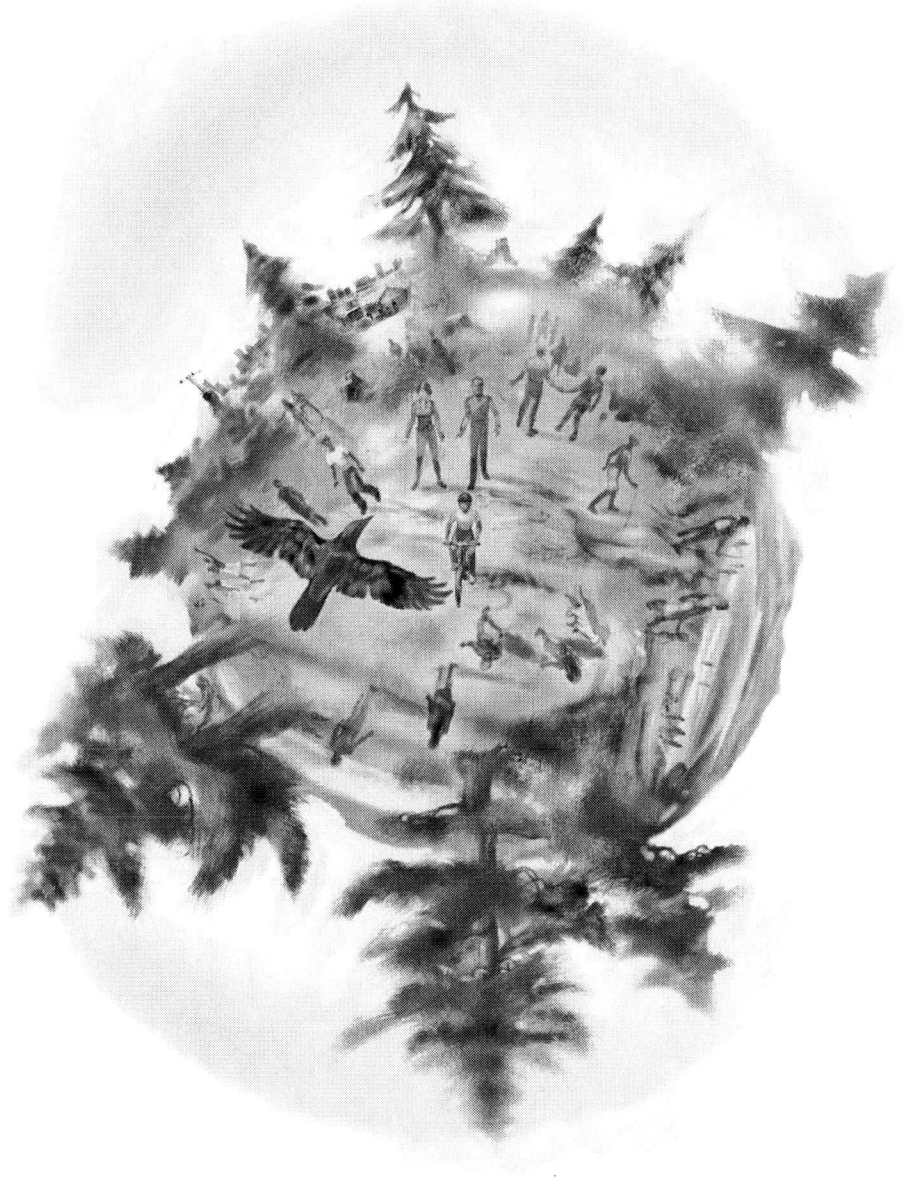

The Sprouted Peanut Vaccine and Other Stories

The Sprouted Peanut Vaccine and Other Stories

Uncrossing Wires

I bump into her for the second time in recent days. She wants me, and lets me know it. I'm attracted to her. Out of habit, I shy away, and nearly go. Then I admit I want her too. She jumps into my arms and lap and I like it.

Now we're outside, near an abandoned garden and house in the countryside. A path goes around the garden. I come up to it from the direction of the house. If I were alone, I'd want to go left, toward a clearing, away from the garden. She goes right, under an arbor, toward a darker area that scares me. I follow her.

We come upon the old compost heap: huge, damp, dark, and fertile. Though abandoned, it has done well. Big, colourful squash are growing near the base. I like the idea they're free. Though not so hungry or into squash these days, I bend down to pick one, then hear buzzing. There must be a wasp's nest near the top of the pile. I move further along the edge of the heap. The path narrows, then meets the woods' edge. I crawl under the young trees' branches to sneak up on the squash without arousing the wasps' suspicion, but a group susses me out. They come buzz right up behind my neck. I'm afraid I'll be stung and it'll hurt and maybe I'll get injured or die.

I'm getting carried away. I've never been allergic to stings. I am not stung.

Emerging from the dream, I feel a pulse of energy at the base of my skull and under the back of my rib cage, followed instantly by a rush of adrenaline. I want to run, fear I can't, and am paralyzed. It's maddening: all pent up and nowhere to go. Is there somewhere I can send the energy? I'm confused. I know I don't need to flee. I start to sweat.

Pulling myself further out of the dream, I feel more surely out of danger. Can I calm the adrenaline somehow? I imagine it spreading out and getting metabolized. At the same time, I blame myself for the strain of such false alarms and worry they may undo some of my progress with the allergy.

I lay awake for a while, wanting both to sleep and to get up. I have a story to tell and the chance to change how I feel about myself. After years of focusing on wounds, new and old, I asked for these dreams and began honing senses. My will to live and sense of purpose grew. Now the visions are coming ever clearer.

I make it out of bed. I feel cold, as the hot adrenaline wears off, and an after-image: I feared that we – Jews, or my mother and I – were going to be attacked; I fled; I find myself safe, but all alone.

It seems I confused son-mother feelings with boyfriend-girlfriend ones; the adrenaline rush of escaping past and death, with the dopamine high of nourishing future and life. Or maybe it's natural that these meet in the present.

I don some warm clothes, have a sip of water, and promise to eat whenever hungry. Nightmares and allergies reveal my hunger for security against an unknown and possibly menacing future, comfort in a difficult moment alone, and sustenance of the journey to which I seem committed. Despite this, I have often deprived myself of food, then binged on it.

I'm not so tired, after all.

The Hypothalamus Who Cried Wolf

"Hey, Hypothalamus!" says Adrenal Gland. "I think I finally got what you were trying to tell me."

"Oh yeah, what's that?" the other replies.

"'Release adrenaline now!'"

Indeed, Hypothalamus (with his pal Pituitary) was pretty darn trigger-happy all those years. Not that it was his fault – doing overtime on guard duty and getting paid, well, peanuts. Unfortunately, Adrenal didn't know that, or was more concerned with his own needs. He tried his best to answer the call, but got worn down and started dragging his feet on the job.

"You freaked me out!" recalls H. T.

"Yeah, so, what did you do? Pushed the button harder!"

"All right, I get the point," H. T. says, pretending to be wounded.

"Ah, don't worry about," says A. G. "You know I missed you."

"So did I."

"The time apart did me good. You don't look so bad yourself."

"Thanks. I'm glad you're back."

A. G. was born to parents who had not much grieved a tragedy. He felt their – and his – lack and pain, and wanted to help. He also wanted the fights to stop. But, ignoring the cause, he didn't know how. And, like them, he sensed that the Big Threat still loomed.

The family of five lived in a big house on a wide street dotted with other big houses whose people too were often away at school or work. Between intense feelings in the boy's body and home, and sparse ones on the surface and outside, a gulf grew. There were few friends or relatives with whom to check in and get comfort. The boy began to cry "help!" seemingly at random.

At first, of course, people rushed to the rescue and he felt secure and even a little mighty. But when they saw no danger, they went away again. The next time he called, they stayed less long. The time after that, they were slower to arrive. And on it went, until others were sent to mind him.

The Sprouted Peanut Vaccine and Other Stories

He felt bad about disturbing them – unable to explain that it wasn't his fault – and because whatever drove him to behave that way still wasn't cured. He missed people twice as much as before! The treatments didn't help and that made things worse. He stopped calling out, reaching instead for sugar, sex, schoolwork, or video games to fill the void. They'd make him feel better for a moment and then worse than before; he'd take more, and get less pleasure and more bad feeling. Even these "good-time" friends were letting him down!

Home was the site of these ills and the ones they sought to appease. Yet, when he had to leave home, he'd rush back as soon as possible. As if to make sure it was still there and its people were okay. And because even a prison can be a familiar home.

Now a young man, he tried going out on his own. The thrill lasted longer and he met people whose ideas, feelings, and activities connected with his, enough so that these could emerge. And how wildly they did! From active to exhausted to renewed and wasted again, he learned about people and things that kindle life, and about the wonder of sometimes doing or having nothing.

Some Things Don't Make Sense

It's snowing buckets. Friday afternoon, off from work, I'm snug in a coffee shop, reading the paper and watching this beloved neighbourhood.

I stop upon a photo of three men, perhaps my age, sitting cross-legged, roadside, wearing headscarves, drinking tea, and gazing downward. One seems lost in his thoughts, or perhaps he is looking at the piece of bread in his hand. The other two look into and beyond their beverages. The caption says, "Migrant Afghani farm workers have their breakfast of hot tea and fresh bread. A peaceful moment in a war-torn country."[246]

It shares the bare-bones feeling of some places I've been in rural West Africa, Native America, and Canada. The flat breads remind me fondly of Tunisian *chapatti* or Indian *naan*.

I have often felt unhealthy eating white bread, and criticized it from the standpoint of nutritional science or concern for the survival of traditional ways. These people can get by, indeed toil, on thin sustenance. Perhaps they will suffer for it later. Meanwhile, here am I, worrying so about eating the right thing, all my life; here are we, in the relatively rich and peaceful countries, with dry goods and fresh produce from around the world, throughout the year, and a booming business of nutritional supplements and "health" foods. What is so demanding about our lives?

When I biked eight hours a day for three weeks across part of the United States, I ate white bread and leftovers and slept in a thin sleeping bag under highway culverts. By living on a dollar a day then, indeed by living below the poverty line most of my adult life, I was only partly trying to live down the material abundance amid which I grew. I was giving form to the affective poverty and stress I felt it came with. Cutting my apprehension of them down to size. Relearning what it feels like to have the space and time to be and relate. Tapping into the happiness of having fewer options and the security of knowing how to function with less.

The poverty I have felt is relative to high expectations of what a child and human should have here. I have been hard on myself and others, yet perhaps all along I have also been generous with them as they have with me – most impressively, when materially "poor."

Sorry I Overreacted

Today is Quebec's national holiday, St. John the Baptist's Day, June 24th. There are street parties everywhere. Around lunch I go to the weekly dance jam; after, we go to the mountain (Montreal's central park) and I give a lesson, listen to some music in another park, and walk home to enjoy a plain dinner alone. Two blocks from my destination, I bump into Katrine, on her way to a block party. "Wanna come?"

It's a beautiful scene. Locals have closed the street and filled it with tables, chairs, couches, carpets, and a band, all with the city's permission. People of all ages and many cultures are standing, dancing, lounging, and having dinner. As soon as we arrive, plates are filled and seats are offered. I know some of these folks casually. The warm welcome feels good and it's hard too, because many days I feel alone and cold, yet aggressed. This past year, especially, I've lost a lot of friends. I was away for a while and living in places where people seemed to take politeness and friendliness more at face-value, less as some come-on or trick.

Afternoon becomes evening and night. *Cumbia* turns to hip-hop, reggaeton, jazz, rock, and at some point a marching samba band. The place goes wild, and peaceful. We don't quit 'til we have to. We clean up and I coast home to bed.

In the morning, I notice the mold and overflowing garbage, and stuff and tense right back up. "What is wrong with these people?" I rail inside. "Even the poorest Third-World family would be ashamed. They act like they don't care, like no one cares about them." From there, it snowballs: the smoking, drinking, staying up late, shabby black clothes, and militant activism. "Why are they killing life!" Do I feel or achieve any differently, living so minimalistically? Would I react so strongly, or at all, if my heart, face, and lungs hadn't so opened last night?

Conclusion

This book began as a challenge to finish curing myself, check that it works for other people, and announce it to the world. But my thoughts and feelings about peanut allergy were already as jumbled as during anaphylaxis, itself, and the extra pressure didn't help.

Today the words that come – for the feeling inside and the understanding developed, from allergy to writing for you – are "good enough." Here's where I'm at.

We who have experienced anaphylaxis aren't categorically distinct from those who haven't, but rather are at one end of a spectrum in which everybody lives somewhere. That spectrum includes asthma, heart palpitations, panic attacks, flashbacks, and other experiences that may be hard to name or connect.

Millions of people in the First World use Ritalin, Prozac, nicotine, alcohol, caffeine, chocolate, sugar, bread, or something else to cope with imbalance somewhere between the extremes of hyperactivity and depression, and excess (allergic) or insufficient immunity. The capacity to go there is brought out in part by living with low-level stress that cannot be escaped, as we are meant to do and can do perhaps more clearly with traditional dangers like war, famine, disease, predators, and extreme weather. Indeed, living relatively free of those dangers can highlight or create low-level stress.

This means that none of us is totally in control of his or her health. That may be scary, but also relieving and useful.

For example, imagine I'm around someone who seems stressed. And say I was stressed to begin with. I may get annoyed at them for adding to my stress, then push them away or try to change them, which probably only makes us both more agitated. Or say I was stressed but am now relieved not to be the only one, and let us both be. If I wasn't stressed to begin with, I might get twice mad at them, for having "made" me stressed. Or, I might be having such a good day, their stress doesn't bother me, and I even feel like doing something to make their life easier.

No matter what my "objective" reality was to start with, how I react can improve or worsen my health and theirs. Shiatsu calls this resonance; psychology calls it empathy. It is going on all the time, in all of our relationships. What enables me to know what you're going through is having felt it, or something like it, at some point in my life. What enables me to help you and learn from you is facing that feeling in myself, while distinguishing what is right for me from what is right for you, especially in this moment.

That said, a certain amount of you "using" me and me "using" you may be natural to surviving and evolving; too much being "nice," a way of not getting involved.

We all have our ways of understanding bodies and feelings. Some traditions see disease as a foreign object or process; others, as a reflection of imbalance. Some wish to suppress symptoms; others, to draw them out. I like a spectral model – from hot to cold, internal to external, male to female, and so on – of bodies, foods, medicines, environments, activities, and relationships, all influencing each other. Here, health is an evolving, imperfect balance, and a process of choice and chance. Therapeutic products and practitioners can help, or not, because they are in relationship with us and the ecology. We can learn how any accessible plant, animal, or inorganic substance affects us, and how that varies with where it comes from, how it's prepared, when it's taken, with what it's taken, and so on.

One disease can be here to heal or prevent another.[247] So maybe somewhere there is a disease that can remedy it. Or maybe the trick is to balance the two, until they cease to threaten or bother life and we call them not disease but natural highs and lows.

In my case, allergy and hyperactivity came at least in part from parental/ancestral trauma, lifestyle, and diet; obsessive-compulsiveness, at least partly as an attempt to reorder those frayed wires; and depression, at least partly to cut the power while doing those repairs. Depression fed constipation, which made things worse, as well as attraction to carbs, sex, exercise, and work, which in cheap form or excess (as addiction) also made things worse but in quality and moderation (as craving) were stepping stones to improvement, in the form a low-protein, active lifestyle. Perhaps one day my nature will have so balanced out that I feel good eating more protein and being less active, or maybe the way I live now will always be right for me; maybe it is even good for people with similar body, ancestry, job, or environment.

Believing that illness is a temporary extreme over which I have some control gives me hope. I practice toning down and tuning up senses, even changing them from pain to pleasure, using the things I need to do everyday, anyway: food, water, activity, rest, eliminating, bathing, and not-eating. These are supported by, and develop, breath, posture, and presence. The results, on the whole, confirm the lifestyle and are transferable from allergy to colds, flus, ear infections, sinus infections, eczema, clogged pores, yeast *(candida)*, athlete's foot, bad breath, heavy body odor, headaches, other aches and pains, irritability, indigestion, bloating, food poisoning, lack of appetite, insatiable appetite, sore joints, bursitis, tendonitis, heart palpitations, cold extremities, overweight, underweight, cuts, bruises, sprains, back pain, shoulder pain, neck stiffness, eye strain, constipation, anxiety, depression, chronic fatigue, and other undiagnosed or undiagnosable conditions. In some cases, herbs, massage, exercises, and other therapies are an added help or necessity. Most of the time it's gradual, with some hard moments and big revelations. It saves me time, money, stress, and side effects, whether from disability, itself, or from the search for someone or something to cure it.

It's amazing what one person can go through, all the while seeming mostly normal. Except for peanut allergy, that is. Or is that, too, changing?

Feedback

"May I speak with Mr. Gottlieb, please?" asks an unfamiliar voice.

"Who's calling?" I bark, having just received one of those calls from a bank trying to interest me in a credit card.

"Ken Dryden."

Oh.

Two weeks ago I e-mailed the successful and conscientious goaltender, author, and minister of parliament, asking for feedback on a draft of this book. Re-reading one of his books, *The Game*, I realized that even as a kid I'd been drawn to the person, not just the star.

After one week, there was no answer. I thought, "this is silly," and gave it one last try.

"Hi, I'm calling to follow up on an e-mail asking Mr. Dryden to review a book of interest to public health. Would it be possible to make an appointment for a short phone call?"

"Are you a friend of his?" she inquired.

"No."

"A constituent?"

"No. Actually, I live in Montreal." (Mr. Dryden's riding is in Toronto.)

Good-naturedly we continued, and left it at that. Later in the week I played ice hockey for the first time ever. Yes, I was a total ice hockey fan and played street hockey every day in the Summer but never did the real thing: wasn't a good skater, didn't want to get hurt, clashed with teammates and opponents, and felt awkward in the locker room. It turns out I'm a natural and the guys (and gals) are great, for the most part.

Mr. Dryden and I talk a while.

When I meet some folks for the first time, it's like I already know and love them, and sometimes it's mutual. Other encounters I don't remember or enjoy as much seem to be able to bring me, and us, there too.

The Sprouted Peanut Vaccine and Other Stories

Dear Family, Friends, and New Acquaintances

I want to make sure you know that, though I do experiment with my allergy and it does change over time, I still check ingredients, eat new foods in small amounts, carry medicine, and tell people about it.

"I've had problems with peanuts. Sometimes severely, other times mildly or not at all. I know, it's funny. It depends on a lot of things. I'm starting to have some good feelings about them. Which I'd like to celebrate with you."

Notes

Introduction

1. In November 2005, in my home province of Québec, fifteen year-old Christina Desforges died of anaphylaxis. She was allergic to peanuts, and had been kissing her boyfriend, who had eaten some of the food earlier in the day. Three months later, the coroner investigating her death announced that she had died of other causes. For an example of how one source changed its story, see 📖 "Girl Dies in Peanut Butter Kiss," *BBC News*, November 29, 2005, *news.bbc.co.uk/ 2/ hi/ americas/ 4481546.stm* and 📖 "Peanut Butter 'Did Not Kill Girl,'" *BBC News*, March 6, 2006, *news.bbc.co.uk/ 2/ hi/ americas/ 4778740.stm*.

   In one study of children known to be at risk of anaphylaxis from eating peanut, none reacted to peanut particles in the air and one-third reacted locally (that is, allergically rather than anaphylactically) to peanut on the skin. 📖 S. H. Sicherer and T. Malloy, *The Complete Peanut Allergy Handbook*, New York: Berkley Books, 2005, pages 142-143.

2. This includes a Bachelor's in Chemistry from Princeton University, Graduate Diploma in Ecotoxicology from Concordia University, and Diploma in Shiatsu Massage Therapy from Guijek Institute. For fifteen years I have been teaching sciences and languages, mostly as a private tutor, with teaching assistanceships at Concordia and the University of Victoria and popular education at various non-profit organizations. For thirteen years, as a volunteer, I produced and hosted public affairs and music programs, on WPRB 103.3 FM Princeton and CKUT 90.3 FM Radio McGill. I have done contracts in many aspects of the food business (service, cooking, farming/gardening, agricultural heritage, and so on) and trained in many arts of physical-emotional wellness (such as aikido, Alexander Technique, Body-Mind Centering®, contact improvisation dance, and yoga).

Allergy, Anaphylaxis, and Intolerance

3. See, for example:

   📖 R. Gupta *et al.*, "Time Trends in Allergic Disorders in the UK," *Thorax*, Volume 62, 2007, pages 91-96.

   📖 F. Rance *et al.*, "Prevalence and Main Characteristics of School Children Diagnosed with Food Allergies in France," *Clinical and Experimental Allergy*, Volume 35, 2005, pages 167-172.

📖 S. H. Sicherer *et al.*, "Prevalence of Peanut and Tree Nut Allergy in the United States Determined by Means of a Random Digit Dial Telephone Survey," *Journal of Allergy and Clinical Immunology*, Volume 112, 2003, pages 1203-1207.

📖 S. L. Taylor and S. L. Helfe, "Update on Food Allergies and Sensitivities," *Food Research Institute Newsletter*, Madison: University of Wisconsin-Madison, Spring 2000.

📖 M. C. Young, *The Peanut Allergy Answer Book*, Gloucester, MA: Fair Winds Press, 2001, pages 21-22.

"First World" is not a universally agreed-upon or accepted term. I take it to mean the community of people living with relatively up-to-date food, health care, sanitation, education, transportation, and other systems. It acknowledges that within a relatively rich country or town there are poor regions and people, and that this may or may not relate to the level of development. I don't mean it to say the First World is better than its counterpart, the "Third World." The terms arose in the mid 1900s, in a context of conflict between much of the First World and a largely communist "Second World." For an example of how these categories are measured today, see 📖 United Nations Development Programme (UNDP), *Human Development Report 2007/2008*, New York: UNDP, 2007, pages 229-232 and 355-359.

[4] 📖 J. van Odijk *et al.*, "Specific IgE Antibodies to Peanut in Western Sweden: Has the Occurrence of Peanut Allergy Increased without an Increase in Consumption?," *Allergy*, Volume 56, 2001, pages 573-577.

[5] 📖 R. K. Woods *et al.*, "International Prevalences of Reported Food Allergies and Intolerances," *European Journal of Clinical Nutrition*, Volume 55, 2001, pages 298-304.

📖 S. A. Bock, "Prospective Appraisal of Complaints of Adverse Reactions to Foods in Children During the First 3 Years of Life," *Pediatrics*, Volume 79, 1987, pages 683-688.

📖 J. J. Niestijl Jansen *et al.*, "Prevalence of Food Allergy and Intolerance in the Adult Dutch Population," *Journal of Allergy and Clinical Immunology*, Volume 93, 1996, pages 446-456.

📖 A. C. Doewes *et al.*, "Prevalentie van Voedselallergie bij Amsterdamse Zuigelingen," *Nederlands Tijdschrift voor Geneeskunde*, Volume 132, 1988, pages 1392-1396.

  📖 Richard Reading, "How Dangerous is Food Allergy in Childhood? The Incidence of Severe and Fatal Allergic Reactions across the UK and Ireland," *Child: Care, Health and Development*, Volume 28, 2002, page 432.

6 📖 Taylor and Helfe, *op. cit.*

7 Non-food allergies seem to be lower there, with exceptions. For example, 📖 R. Beasley, "Worldwide Variation in Prevalence of Symptoms of Asthma, Allergic Rhinoconjunctivitis, and Atopic Eczema: ISAAC," *Lancet*, Volume 351, 1998, pages 1225-1232, found that asthma was highest in the British Isles and Australia-New Zealand, followed by the Americas; asthma, *eczema* (a collection of skin irritation symptoms), and *rhinoconjunctivitis* (a collection of ear, nose, and/or throat irritation symptoms) were lowest in Eastern Europe, Central and Southeast Asia, and Eastern Africa, with some high-eczema zones in Northern Europe and Africa. In general, these diseases have been rising for decades in the First World.

  See also 📖 R. Polosa, "Prevalence of Atopy and Urban Air Pollution: Dirty Business," *Clinical and Experimental Allergy*, Volume 29, 1999, pages 1439-1441.

8 📖 Sicherer and Malloy, *op. cit.*, page 131.

  📖 M. Wensing *et al.*, "The Distribution of Individual Threshold Doses Eliciting Allergic Reactions in a Population with Peanut Allergy," *Journal of Allergy and Clinical Immunology*, Volume 110, 2002, pages 915-920.

  📖 Young, *op. cit.*, pages 48-49.

9 📖 Agency for Healthcare Research and Quality, "Treatment Costs Nearly Double for Hay Fever and Other Allergies," *AHRQ News and Numbers*, June 11, 2008, *www.ahrq.gov/ news/ nn/ nn061108.htm*. Spending was measured in 2005 and 2000.

  📖 Kalorama Information, *The U.S. Market for Over-the-Counter Allergy and Asthma Products*, Rockville, MD: Market Research.com, 2001. Spending was measured in 2000.

10 📖 M. J. Weiss, "The Season for Sneezin'," *American Demographics*, Volume 13, 1999, page *.

11 📖 J. Buttriss, "Food Allergy and Intolerance: What are the Facts?," *Student British Medical Journal*, Volume 9, 2001, pages 357-398.

12 There can be many other symptoms, such as vomiting, diarrhea, dizziness, and uterine contractions. 📖 Sicherer and Malloy, *op. cit.*, pages 258-259.

[13] For this and other endeavours, Richet was awarded the 1913 Nobel Prize in Physiology and Medicine. 📖 J. A. Simpson and E. S. C. Weiner, eds., *The Oxford English Dictionary*, Oxford: Clarendon, Volume 1, pages 334 and 437.

[14] 📖 F. N. Kotsonis et al., "Food Toxicology," *Casarett and Doull's Toxicology*, New York: McGraw-Hill, 1996, pages 909-949.

[15] 📖 D. Nambudripad, NAET: *Say Good-Bye to Your Allergies,* Buena Park, CA: Delta Publishing, 2003, page 7.

[16] 📖 B. Katzung, "Drugs with Important Actions on Smooth Muscle: Histamine, Serotonin, and the Ergot Alkaloids," *Basic and Clinical Pharmacology*, New York: McGraw-Hill, 2004, pages 259-280.

📖 M. L. Foegh and P. W. Ramwell, "The Eicosanoids: Prostaglandins, Thromboxanes, Leukotrienes, and Related Compounds," *Basic and Clinical Pharmacology*, New York: McGraw-Hill, 2004, pages 298-312.

📖 P. Fireman, "The Mechanisms of Allergic Inflammation: Anaphylaxis Described," *Discover*, Volume 20, 1999, pages S16-S19, supplement to Issue 3.

Some sources don't consider thromboxanes to be inflammatory in the same sense as the other two.

[17] All of our proteins come from various combinations of 20 *alpha* amino acids. Ten of these we can make aplenty, and ten we have to get totally or partly from food. For this reason, the latter group is said to be *essential*. Histidine is essential, at least in children.

[18] 📖 R. Wyatt, "Anaphylaxis: How to Recognize, Treat, and Prevent Potentially Fatal Attacks," *Postgraduate Medicine*, Volume 100, 1996, pages 87-99.

📖 Sicherer and Malloy, page 108.

[19] About a four-to-one proportion of adrenaline and noradrenaline is sent. They have similar effects, and collaborate to raise blood pressure: adrenaline is the stronger heartrate stimulator; noradrenaline is the stronger blood vessel constrictor.

[20] 📖 M. Jackson, *Allergy: The History of a Modern Malady*, London: Reaktion, 2006, page 28.

📖 Young, *op. cit.*, page 20.

[21] 📖 S. A. Bock, "The Natural History of Food Sensitivity," *Journal of Allergy and Clinical Immunology*, Volume 69, 1982, pages 173-177.

📖 S. A. Bock and F. M. Atkins, "The Natural History of Peanut Allergy," *Journal of Allergy and Clinical Immunology*, Volume 83, 1989, pages 900-904.

[22] 📖 H. S. Skolnick et al., "The Natural History of Peanut Allergy," *Journal of Allergy and Clinical Immunology*, Volume 107, 2001, pages 367-374.

📖 J. O.'B. Hourihane et al., "Resolution of Peanut Allergy: Case-Control Study," *British Medical Journal*, Volume 316, 1998, pages 1271-1275.

📖 J. M. Spergel et al., "Natural History of Peanut Allergy," *Current Opinion in Pediatrics*, Volume 13, 2001, pages 517-522.

[23] 📖 T. David, "Patients Have Not Been Proved to Grow out of Peanut Allergy," *British Medical Journal*, Volume 317, 1998, page 1317.

[24] 📖 D. M. Fleischer et al., "The Natural Progression of Peanut Allergy: Resolution and the Possibility of Recurrence," *Journal of Allergy and Clinical Immunology*, Volume 112, 2003, pages 183-189.

📖 J. M. Spergel et al., "Resolution of Childhood Peanut Allergy," *Annals of Allergy, Asthma, and Immunology*, Volume 85, 2000, pages 473-476.

📖 D. M. Fleischer, "Peanut Allergy: Recurrence and Its Management," *Journal of Allergy and Clinical Immunology*, Volume 114, 2004, pages 1195-1201.

[25] 📖 Young, *op. cit.*, pages 90-91, cites one medical report from the 1930s and others starting in the 1980s.

[26] Current practitioners who have published their methods include 📖 Nambudripad, *op. cit.* and 📖 E. Cutler, *The Food Allergy Cure*, New York: Three Rivers Press, 2003.

Fasciatherapy works to release tension held in the thin membranes, including the one that envelops the whole body, just below the skin, and those that surround muscles or hold soft organs in place. Muscle testing *(kinesiology)* is a chiropractic approach to the anatomy of movement, and, among other things, treats the nerves that run through muscles.

[27] 📖 L. Pons et al., "Towards Immunotherapy for Peanut Allergy," *Current Opinion in Allergy and Clinical Immunology*, Volume 5, 2005, pages 558-562.

📖 X.-M. Li, "Beyond Allergen Avoidance: Update on Developing Therapies for Peanut Allergy," *Current Opinion in Allergy and Clinical Immunology*, Volume 5, 2005, pages 287-292.

📖 K. D. Srivastava et al., "The Chinese Herbal Medicine Formula FAHF-2 Completely Blocks Anaphylactic Reactions in a Murine Model of Peanut Allergy," *Journal of Allergy and Clinical Immunology*, Volume 115, 2005, pages 171-178. In this study, peanut-allergic mice were treated with FAHF-2 for 7 weeks, then fed peanut meal 1, 3, and 5 weeks afterwards. None of them had anaphylaxis, while all of their untreated peers did. The formula is 20 parts reishi mushroom *(ling zhi)*, 20 parts *mume* fruit *(wu mei)*, 6 parts coptis root *(huang lian)*, 6 parts ginger root *(gan jiang)*, 6 parts ginseng root *(ren shen)*, 6 parts Chinese angelica root *(dang gui)*, 4 parts *huang bai* root, 2 parts cinnamon twig *(gui zhi)*, and 1 part Szechuan pepper seed *(chuan jiao)*.

[28] 📖 J. O.'B. Hourihane et al., "Resolution of Peanut Allergy Following Bone Marrow Transplantation for Primary Immunodeficiency," *Allergy*, Volume 60, 2005, pages 536-537.

[29] For example, there is breeding to alter protein and reduce aflatoxin. 📖 H. Dodo et al., "A Genetic Engineering Strategy to Eliminate Peanut Allergy," *Current Allergy and Asthma Reports*, Volume 5, 2005, pages 67-73. 📖 P. Wesche-Ebeling et al., "Food and Feed Science," *The Peanut (Arachis Hypogaea) Crop*, Enfield, NH: Science Publishers, 2002, page 274. These and other potential causes of allergy are discussed in a few chapters' time.

Irradiation is another strategy being tried for some other allergenic foods. 📖 M.-W. Byun et al., "Application of Gamma Irradiation for Inhibition of Food Allergy," *Radiation Physics and Chemistry*, Volume 63, 2002, pages 369-370.

[30] 📖 Sicherer and Malloy, *op. cit.*, pages 49 and 67-68.

📖 Young, *op. cit.*, pages 10-14.

📖 A. T. Clark and P. W. Ewan, "Interpretation of Tests for Nut Allergy in One Thousand Patients, in Relation to Allergy or Tolerance," *Clinical and Experimental Allergy*, Volume 33, 2003, pages 1019-1022.

📖 J. K. Kishiyama, "Allergic & Immunologic Disorders" in L. M. Tierney *et al.*, eds., *Current Medical Diagnosis and Treatment*, New York: Lange, 2006, pages 788-806.

A Gift

[31] 🎧 H. Michel, interview by A. Gottlieb, "AIDS Awareness: A Personal Account," *Native Solidarity News*, Episode 218, 2000, first broadcast on CKUT 90.3 FM Radio McGill.

Who's a Nut?

[32] 📖 R. K. Maiti, "About the Peanut Crop," *The Peanut (Arachis Hypogaea) Crop*, Enfield, NH: Science Publishers, 2002, pages 1-7.

33 📖 R. K. Maiti and P. Wesche-Ebeling, "Vegetative, Reproductive Growth and Productivity," *The Peanut (Arachis Hypogaea) Crop*, Enfield, NH: Science Publishers, 2002, pages 73-96.

34 Nuts come from various families. For example, walnuts and pecans are related to hickory, almonds are related to apples and peaches (and roses), and cashews and pistachios are related to mangoes (and poison ivy).

35 📖 R. K. Maiti and P. Wesche-Ebeling, "Seeds, Germination and Crop Establishment," *The Peanut (Arachis Hypogaea) Crop*, Enfield, NH: Science Publishers, 2002, pages 31-50.

 📖 R. K. Maiti et al. "Root System and Mineral Nutrition," *The Peanut (Arachis Hypogaea) Crop*, Enfield, NH: Science Publishers, 2002, page 144.

36 📖 A. F. Smith, *Peanuts: The Illustrious History of the Goober Pea*, Urbana: University of Illinois Press, 2002, pages 1-19.

37 Numbers 1, 2, 3, and 5 are soy, canola, cotton, and sunflower, respectively. 📖 Food and Agriculture Organization of the United Nations, "Oilseeds, Oils and Oilmeals," *FAO Outlook*, December 2006, page 19.

38 📖 Maiti, *op. cit.*

39 Some of the symptoms noted were headache, dizziness, and indigestion. In the early 1900s, just before their mass-popularization, peanuts suddenly became fashionable among wealthy Americans. 📖 Smith, *op. cit.*, pages 1-19 and 30-44.

40 📖 Young, *op. cit.*, page 19.

 📖 Smith, *op. cit.*, pages 36 and 132.

 📖 H. Boriss and M. Kreith, *Commodity Profile: Peanuts*, Davis, CA: University of California Agricultural Issues Center, 2006.

 📖 United States Department of Agriculture, "Peanut Consumption Rebounding Amidst Market Uncertainties," *Agricultural* Outlook, March 2002, pages 2-5. 📖 United States Department of Commerce, "Roasted Nuts and Peanut Butter Manufacturing: 2002," *2002 Economic Census*, December 2004.

41 📖 Jackson, *op. cit.*, page 146.

Peanut Butter to the Rescue!

42 📖 Smith, *op. cit.*, pages 1-44 and 101-120.

📖 United States Census Bureau, *Historical National Population Estimates: July 1, 1900 to July 1, 1999*, 2000, www.census.gov/ popest/ archives/ 1990s/ popclockest.txt.

Half of *Oh Henry!*'s 1943 record-breaking sales went to the army. *Snickers*, introduced by Ethel Mars in 1930, remains the best-selling bar in the world.

Why Peanuts?

43 Compare, for example, 📖 D. Barnett *et al.*, "Multiplicity of Allergens in Peanuts," *Journal of Allergy and Clinical Immunology*, Volume 72, 1983, pages 61-68, with 📖 Young, *op. cit.*, pages 48-49.

44 📖 Cutler, *op. cit.*

   📖 Nambudripad, *op. cit.*

45 📖 Young, *op. cit.*, page 27.

46 Its name comes from the Latin word for peanut, *arachis*.

47 Another way of saying this is that they are relatively acidic, and disrupt the body's acid-alkaline balance. In contrast, the *linoleic* and *linolenic* fatty acids that dominate in many foods produce metabolites that tend to alkalize and clean the body and favour long-term health. This includes PGE_1, PGE_3, and the PGE_3 precursors known as *omega-3* fatty acids. Arachidonic acid also has many benefits and vital roles, for example in maintaining a healthy central nervous system. 📖 P. Pitchford, *Healing with Whole Foods*, Berkeley: North Atlantic Books, 1993, pages 133-134.

48 📖 A. Ber, "Neutralization of Phenolic (Aromatic) Food Compounds in a Holistic General Practice," *Journal of Orthomolecular Psychiatry*, Volume 12, 1983, pages 283-291.

   Clearing for phenolics – getting a person used to them, so that they no longer react – is part of one peanut allergy treatment. 📖 Cutler, *op. cit.*, page 70.

49 📖 Cutler, *op. cit.*, page 72.

50 These are in the *aspergillus* family, which includes molds used to make foods and drinks like soy sauce and *sake* (Japanese rice alcohol).

   The concentration may be particularly high in peanut skin and peanut butter. 📖 Smith, *op. cit.*, pages 118-119. 📖 M. R. Paulsen *et al.*, "Aflatoxin Content and Skin Removal of Spanish Peanuts as Affected by Treatments with Chemicals, Water Spray, Heated Air, and Liquid Nitrogen". *Journal of Food Science*, Volume 41, 1976, pages 667–71.

51   📖 P. Wesche-Ebeling *et al.*, *op. cit.*.

52   Another example is allergy to eggs and milk during ragweed pollen season. 📖 Cutler, *op. cit.*, page 30.

53   More completely: vata is typified by a tall and thin body, dry skin, nervous disposition, and active lifestyle; pitta, by a muscular build, moist and reddish skin, tendency to fever and inflammation, and competitiveness; and kapha, by a full body, thick and oily skin, vulnerability to congestive illness, and professional steadiness. Everybody is some mix of these three humours (*doshas*). The mix may be different in physical and emotional areas, and changes over time.

Illnesses are linked to excess or deficiency of particular doshas, and healed by moderating them as well as by reinforcing or toning down complementary doshas. For example, high blood pressure reflects high pitta, is aggravated by fiery foods and emotions, and is soothed by watery or airy ones.

That said, a food's energetic quality can be changed somewhat by how it is prepared. For example, dry roasting peanuts makes them even more pitta, but sprouting makes them more kapha and thus suitable to pitta-vata people. 📖 D. Frawley, *Ayurvedic Healing*, Twin Lakes, WI: Lotus Press, 2000, pages 29-41.

54   In the United States, the practice grew in part from the need to combat pests to the lucrative cotton crop and restore nutrients it takes from the soil. 📖 K. P. Paudel *et al.*, "Economic and Environmental Evaluations of Peanut Rotations with Switchgrass and Cotton," *Highlights of Agricultural Research*, Volume 43, 1996, pages 4-7.

Another rotation example is peanut with millet or sorghum cereal, in West Africa. 📖 R. K. Maiti *et al.*, "Agronomy and Productivity," *The Peanut (Arachis Hypogaea) Crop*, Enfield, NH: Science Publishers, 2002, pages 70-71.

55   See, for example, 📖 H. R. Newsome *et al.*, "Pesticide Residues in the Canadian Market Based Survey: 1992 to 1996," *Food Additives and Contaminants*, Volume 17, 2000, pages 847–54. Among foods surveyed and representing 99% of a typical Canadian diet, butter and peanut butter were highest in pesticide residues.

56   There is a whole spectrum: from the farmer or researcher who saves the seeds of an individual plant remarkable for its productivity, disease resistance, food quality, shelf life, or ease of shipping and processing; to the one who hybridizes that plant with a related species, to improve any of those features; to the researcher who submits cells of that plant to shocks that

produce various mutations, until they find one that is useful; to the one who splices the genes of such a cell with those of another, to specifically change some property. The latter seems to be what many people associate with "genetic engineering."

57 📖 E. Barnes, *Diseases and Human Evolution*, Albuquerque: University of New Mexico Press, page 315.

58 Some of the common additives include partially hydrogenated vegetable oil, sugar, and maltodextrin (a sweetener made from corn, potato, rice, or other starch).

59 📖 Young, *op. cit.*, pages 86-87.

60 Radiation is at once a substance and pure energy. The most intense forms are *alpha, beta,* and *gamma* nuclear fallout, X-rays, and ultraviolet (UV) light. After that come visible light, infrared (IR), microwaves, and radio. Higher energy often means more radical perturbation of cells and systems; however, microwave ovens, cell phone radio waves, extremely low frequency (ELF) fields from power lines and electrical appliances, and natural magnetic storms may also have effects. 📖 World Health Organization, *Electromagnetic Fields*, fact sheets 299, 304, and 322, Geneva: World Health Organization, 2006-2007.

61 📖 Nambudripad, *op. cit.*, page 4.

62 According to 📖 Barnes, *op. cit.*, pages 417-418, it was only in the early 1970s, with a rise in energy prices and consequent need to save energy, that such closed environments – and asthma – proliferated.

63 This has been called the "hygiene hypothesis." 📖 Sicherer and Malloy, *op. cit.*, pages 12-13.

64 Other functions include recycling red blood cells, making blood proteins, storing emergency reserves of blood and sugar-energy *(glycogen)*, and storing and releasing the fat-soluble vitamins A, D, E, and K. 📖 L. Ide, *Anatomie des systèmes*, Montreal: Guijek, 2004, pages 41-42.

65 Lymphatic vessels traverse the body, often close to the blood vessels, from whose smallest branches *(capillaries)* the lymph fluid absorbs toxins. When the fluid gets to the nodes, it is filtered and treated with immune cells *(lymphocytes)*, before reentering contact with the blood. This protects the heart and downstream organs, but can inflame the nodes. 📖 S. Romagnani, "The Role of Lymphocytes in Allergic Disease," *Journal of Allergy and Clinical Immunology*, Volume 105, 2000, pages 399-408. 📖 Characterization of Lymphocyte Responses to Peanuts in Normal Children, Peanut-Allergic

Children, and Allergic Children Who Acquired Tolerance to Peanuts," *Journal of Clinical Investigation*, Volume 111, 2003, pages 1065-1072.

The Peanut Detective Squad

66   S. L. Taylor *et al.*, "Food Allergies and Sensitivities" in S. L. Taylor and R. A. Scanlan, ed., *Food Toxicology: A Perspective on the Relative Risks*, New York: Dekker, 1989, pages 255-295.

Young, *op. cit.*, page 41.

S. C. Dreskin and G. W. Palmer, "Anaphylaxis," *e-Medicine*, 2005, *www.emedicine.com/ med/ topic128.htm*.

Health Canada, *Food Allergies*, 2007, *www.hc-sc.gc.ca/ fn-an/ securit/ allerg/ fa-aa/ index-eng.php*.

67   J. O.'B. Hourihane *et al.*, "An Evaluation of the Sensitivity of Subjects with Peanut Allergy to Very Low Doses of Peanut Protein: A Randomize, Double-Blind, Placebo-Controlled Food Challenge Study," *Journal of Allergy and Clinical Immunology*, Volume 100, 1997, pages 596-600. Systemic and non-systemic reactions were found at doses as low as 0.005 grams.

J. Strid *et al.*, "A Novel Model of Sensitization and Oral Tolerance to Peanut Protein," *Immunology*, Volume 113, 2004, pages 293-303.

68   J. A. Nordlee *et al.*, "Allergenicity of Various Peanut Products as Determined by RAST Inhibition," *Journal of Allergy and Clinical immunology*, Volume 68, 1981, pages 376-382.

69   Nutrition Data, *www.nutritiondata.com*.

70   University of Texas Medical Branch, "Structural Database of Allergenic Proteins," *fermi.utmb.edu/ SDAP /index.html*.

71   D. L. Buchhagen, "Limiting C Damage," *Journal of Immunology* Volume 174, 2005, pages 1-2.

72   T. S. Kholief, "Chemical Composition and Protein Properties of Peanuts," *Zeitschrift fur Ernährungswissenschaft*, Volume 26, 1987, pages 56-51.

Nutrition Data, *op. cit.*

73   S. Y. Chung *et al.*, "Linking Peanut Allergenicity to the Process of Maturation, Curing, and Roasting," *Journal of Agricultural and Food Chemistry*, Volume 51, 2003, pages 4273-4277.

Over 90% of US food peanuts are dry roasted, whether for use in peanut butter or sale in or out of shell. 📖 S. Sanford, "U.S. Peanut Consumption Rebounds," *United States Department of Agriculture Agricultural Outlook,* December 1998, pages 12-15.

74 📖 G. Lack *et al.*, "Factors Associated with the Development of Peanut Allergy in Childhood," *New England Journal of Medicine,* Volume 348, 2003, pages 977-985.

75 📖 Pitchford, *op. cit.*, page 138. Food oils are a mixture of fats known as saturates, monounsaturates, and polyunsaturates, depending on how many reactive carbon-carbon bonds they have. Arachidonic acid is a 20-carbon polyunsaturate. The reactive sites can be filled (*saturated*) by processes such as hydrogenation and make free radicals or polymers, for example when cooked or refined at a high temperature. The relative stability of saturates makes them harder to metabolize but safe from those dangers. Perhaps for this reason, monounsaturates, which dominate in olive and oleic oils, may be touted as healthiest or most balanced.

76 💻 Nutrition Data, *op cit.*

77 This is canola that has been bred to have more monounsaturates and less polyunsaturates than other varieties. Canola is also known as rapeseed.

78 💻 J. Weisnagel, "Peanut Allergy: Where Do We Stand?" Association of Allergists and Immunologists of Quebec, *www.allerg.qc.ca/ peanutallergy.htm#oil.*

79 Most peanut oil sold in the First World is of the latter kind. 📖 Young, *op. cit.,* page 61. 📖 Taylor and Helfe, *op. cit.* 📖 Sicherer and Malloy, *op. cit.*, page 167.

80 📖 Pitchford, *op. cit.*, pages 132 and 328. Foods lower in arachidonic acid include grains, legumes, other nuts, seeds, fruit, vegetables, mother's milk, organ meats, and fish.

81 💻 V. Crump, "Prognosis of Severe Food Allergies," 2002, Auckland Allergy Clinic, *www.allergyclinic.co.nz/ guides/ 45.html.*

82 📖 Cutler, *op. cit.*

  📖 Ber, *op. cit.*

83 The onion family includes plants like onions, leeks, chives, garlic, and asparagus, while nightshades include eggplant, peppers, potato, and tomato.

84 📖 Ber, *op. cit.*

85   The Cleveland Clinic, "Special Diets for Food Allergies," www.clevelandclinic.org/ health/ health-info/ docs/ 2900/ 2987.asp?index= 10014.

86   Auckland Allergy Clinic, "Salicylate Sensitivity," 2001, www.allergyclinic.co.nz/ guides/ 30.html.

87   Allergy Clinics of London, "Food Allergy and Addictive Intolerance," www.allergyhospital.co.uk/ food_ allergy_ for_ doctors.htm.

88   S. A. Miller, "Food Additives and Contaminants," *Casarett and Doull's Toxicology*, New York: McGraw-Hill, 1991, pages 846-847.

J. A. DiPaolo et al., "Teratogenic Response by Hamsters, Rats and Mice to Aflatoxin B_1," *Nature*, Volume 215, 1967, pages 638-639.

Wesche-Ebeling, op. cit., page 268.

89   A 1958 epidemic of sudden death among UK turkeys fed contaminated peanut meal helped identify the aflatoxin risk. H. Fonseca, "Fungal Toxins Found in Foods," *Micotoxinas Boletim*, Number 27, www.micotoxinas.com.br/ boletim27.htm. See also:

K. Sergeant et al., "Toxicity Associated with Certain Samples of Groundnuts," *Nature*, Volume 192, 1961, pages 1096-1097.

U. L. Diener et al., "Toxin-Producing *Aspergillus* Isolated from Domestic Peanuts," *Science*, Volume 142, 1963, pages 1491-1492.

Z. Cope, "Carcinogens in Groundnuts," *British Medical Journal*, Volume 2, 1964, pages 204-205.

90   C. Wilson, "Mold Allergy: Facts and Treatment," Asheville, NC: Great Smokies Medical Center, www.gsmcweb.com/ www/ html%20pages/ mold%20allergy%20print.htm.

Auckland Allergy Clinic, "Allergy Prevention," Guide 27, www.allergyclinic.co.nz/ guides/ 27.html.

United States Department of Health and Human Services, "Cigarette Smoke Makes Allergy Symptoms Worse" www.healthfinder.gov/ newsletters/ allergy071706. asp#701965.

91   F. Waliyar, *Managing Aflatoxin in Groundnut*, Patancheru, India: International Crops Research Institute for the Semi-Arid Tropics, 2008, www.aflatoxin.info/ maig.asp.

92   G. E. Piérard et al., "Comparative Clinicopathological Manifestations of Human Aspergillosis," *Exogenous Dermatology*, Volume 3, 2004, pages 144-153.

93 H. S. Black, "Mechanisms of Pro- and Antioxidation," *Journal of Nutrition*, Volume 134, 2004, pages 3169S-3170S.

94 Young, *op. cit.*, pages 30-31.

95 Sicherer and Malloy, *op. cit.*, page 32.

96 D. Mittag *et al.*, "Birch Pollen-Related Food Allergy to Legumes," *Clinical and Experimental Allergy*, Volume 35, 2005, page 1049.

 L. V. Crawford *et al.*, "Immunologic Studies on the Legume Family of Foods," *Annals of Allergy*, Volume 23, 1965, pages 303-308.

97 Young, *op. cit.*, pages 31-32. In the same survey, many people with peanut allergy also report being allergic to milk and fish/shellfish.

98 Allergy/Asthma Information Association, "Peanut Allergy," *www.aaia.ca/english/ articles/ pdf/ aaia_ peanut_ allergy_ brochure2pg.pdf.*

99 Sicherer and Malloy, *op. cit.*, page 34.

100 R. Pumphrey, "Peanuts and Panic: Coping with Anaphylaxis," DotPharmacy, *www.dotpharmacy.co.uk/ upnuts.html.*

101 M. Rachmiel *et al.*, "The Importance of the Pecan Tree Pollen in Allergic Manifestations," *Clinical and Experimental Allergy*, Volume 26, 1996, pages 323-329.

 American Academy of Allergy, Asthma and Immunology, "Food Allergy," 2005, *www.aaaai.org/ AADMC/ ate/ category.asp?cat=1057&s=40&keywords=.*

102 D. F. Gibb, "Anaphylaxis from Pollen Introduced by a Bee Sting," *Canadian Medical Association Journal*, Volume 19, 1928, page 461.

103 Cutler, *op. cit.*, page 29.

 M. Rottem and Y. Waisel, "Food Allergy to Concealed Sunflower Pollen," *Allergy*, Volume 53, 1998, pages 719-720.

104 D. Mittag *et al.*, "Ara h 8, a Bet v 1-Homologous Allergen from Peanut, Is a Major Allergen in Patients with Combined Birch Pollen and Peanut Allergy," *Journal of Allergy and Clinical Immunology*, Volume 114, 2004, 1410-1417.

 C. G. Mortz *et al.*, "The Prevalence of Peanut Sensitizations and the Association to Pollen Sensitization in a Cohort of Unselected Adolescents – the Odense Adolescence Cohort Study on Atopic Diseases and Dermatitis (TOACS)," *Pediatric Allergy and Immunology*, Volume 16, 2005, pages 501-506.

105 For example, birch pollen has been linked to almond, brazil nut, hazelnut, walnut, apple, cherry, peach, plum, carrot, and potato allergies. 📖 W.-H. Boehncke et al., "Identification of HLA-DR and -DQ Alleles Conferring Susceptibility to Pollen Allergy and Pollen Associated Food Allergy," *Clinical and Experimental Allergy*, Volume 28, 1998, pages 434-441.

📖 N. E. Eriksson et al., "Food Hypersensitivity in Patients with Pollen Allergy," *Allergy*, Volume 37, 1982, pages 437-443.

📖 Mittag et al., op. cit.

106 📖 H. Breiteneder et al., "The Gene Coding for the Major Birch Pollen Allergen betv1, Is Highly Homologous to a Pea Disease Resistance Response Gene," *EMBO Journal*, Volume 8, 1989, pages 1935-1938.

107 💻 Mayo Clinic Staff, "Peanut Allergy," *www.mayoclinic.com/ health/ peanut-allergy/ DS00710/ DSECTION=4*.

108 📖 S. H. Sicherer et al., "Genetics of Peanut Allergy: A Twin Study," *Journal of Allergy and Clinical Immunology*, Volume 106, 2000, pages 53-56.

📖 J. O.'B. Hourihane et al., "Peanut Allergy in Relation to Heredity, Maternal Diet, and Other Atopic Diseases: Results of a Questionnaire Survey, Skin Prick Testing, and Food Challenges," *British Medical Journal*, Volume 313, 1996, pages 518-521. In this study, parents were also slightly more likely to share peanut allergy, while grandparents, aunts, and uncles were not.

109 See, for example, 📖 P. J. Hannaway et al., "Differences in Race, Ethnicity, and Socioeconomic Status in Schoolchildren Dispensed Injectable Epinephrine in 3 Massachusetts School Districts," *Annals of Allergy, Asthma, and Immunology*, Volume 95, 2005, pages 143-148.

110 💻 United States Agricultural Research Service, "Identification and Characterization of Genes Important During Seed Development in Legumes," 2006, *www.ars.usda.gov/ research/ projects/ projects.htm? ACCN_NO= 410458&fy= 2006*.

111 See, for example, 📖 M. M. Amoli et al., "Polymorphism in the STAT6 Gene Encodes Risk for Nut Allergy," *Genes and Immunity*, Volume 3, 2002, pages 220-224.

112 💻 Pesticide Action Network, "Pesticides Database" *www.pesticideinfo.org*.

📖 C. Swadener, "Bacillus thuringiensis Insecticide Fact Sheet" *Journal of Pesticide Reform* Volume 14, 1994.

As of at least 2003, genetically modified peanuts containing Bt have been experimented with but not sold in the US, and Bt spray has not usually been used on peanut crops. 💻 University of Florida Institute of Food and Agricultural Science, *edis.ifas.efl.edu*.

[113] 💻 Massachusetts Department of Agricultural Resources, "Groundwater Protection List Details" *www.mass.gov/ agr/ pesticides/ water/ groundwater%20 protection%20 list% details% for%20 web% site%202.0.htm*.

📖 United States Environmental Protection Agency, "Dioxin: Scientific Highlights from the NAS Review Draft of EPA's Dioxin Reassessment" October 15, 2004.

[114] Propargite is an insecticide that impairs the ATP *(adenosine triphosphate)* energy cycle in spider mites; human health effects include skin and eye irritation and intestinal cancer. Methyl parathion is a stomach poison to worms that prey on cotton plant; in humans it especially perturbs the central nervous system and liver. 💻 United States Centers for Disease Control and Prevention, "Agents, Diseases, and Other Threats," *www.bt.cdc.gov/ agent*.

📖 D. K. Ecobichon, "Toxic Effects of Pesticides," *Casarett and Doull's Toxicology*, New York: McGraw-Hill, 1991, pages 565-622.

[115] 💻 Pesticide Action Network, *op. cit.*

[116] 💻 United States Department of Agriculture, "Petitions of Nonregulated Status Granted or Pending by Aphis as of 24 July 2008," *www.aphis.usda.gov/ brs/ not_reg.html*.

[117] 📖 V. Nagarajan and R. V. Bhat, "Aflatoxin Production in Peanut Varieties by *Aspergillus Flavus* Link and *Aspergillus Parasiticus* Speare," *Applied Microbiology*, Volume 25, 1973, pages 319-321.

📖 S. J. Koppelman *et al.*, "Quantification of Major Peanut Allergens Ara h 1 and Ara h 2 in the Peanut Varieties Runner, Spanish, Virginia, and Valencia, Bred in Different Parts of the World," *Allergy*, Volume 56, 2001, pages 132-137.

[118] 📖 Wesche-Ebeling *et al.*, *op. cit.*, pages 245-256.

[119] 📖 A. Layrisse *et al.*, "Combining Ability for Yield, Protein and Oil of Peanut Lines from South American Centers of Diversity," *Euphytica*, Volume 29, 1980, pages 561-570.

💻 United States Department of Agriculture, *op. cit.*

[120] 📖 J. F. Eheart *et al.*, "Variety, Type, Year, and Location Effects on the Chemical Composition of Peanuts," *Food Research*, Volume 20, 1955, pages 497-505.

📖 M. Luo *et al.*, "Microarray-Based Screening of Differentially Expressed Genes in Peanut in Response to Aspergillus Parasiticus Infection and Drought Stress," *Plant Science*, Volume 169, 2005, pages 695-703

[121] Produce may be irradiated to kill microbes, insects, and other organisms that can harm local crops or consumers, as well as to delay ripening, prevent sprouting, and have other effects. It can be voluntary or required by law, and imported and domestic produce may be treated differently.

[122] 📖 M. C. van Putten *et al.*, "Novel Foods and Food Allergies: A Review of the Issues," *Trends in Food Science and Technology*, Volume 17, 2006, pages 289-299.

[123] See, for example, 📖 Jackson, *op. cit.*, page 174, about a Saudi Arabian study on returning to typical rural foods.

[124] 📖 Luo *et al.*, *op. cit.*

📖 Chung *et al.*, *op. cit.*

[125] 📖 Strid *et al.*, *op. cit.*

[126] 📖 van Putten *et al.*, *op cit*.

[127] 📖 S. Sicherer *et al.*, "Clinical Features of Acute Allergic Reactions to Peanut and Tree Nuts in Children," *Pediatrics*, Volume 102, 1998, page e6.

[128] 📖 Sicherer and Malloy, *op. cit.*, pages 21-22.

[129] 📖 J. Strid *et al.*, "Epicutaneous Exposure to Peanut Protein Prevents Oral Tolerance and Enhances Allergic Sensitization," *Clinical and Experimental Allergy*, Volume 35, 2005, pages 757-766.

[130] 📖 Strid *et al.*, *op. cit.* (2004).

[131] 📖 D. Leung and S. Bock, "Progress in Peanut Allergy Research: Are We Closer to a Cure?," *Journal of Allergy and Clinical Immunology*, Volume 112, 2003, pages 112-114.

📖 B. Niggemann *et al.*, "Specific IgE Levels Do Not Indicate Persistence or Transience of Food Allergy in Children with Atopic Dermatitis," *Journal of Investigative Allergology and Clinical Immunology*, Volume 14, 2004, pages 98-103.

[132] 📖 Fleischer *et al.*, *op. cit.* (2004). See also note 21.

[133] 📖 Hourihane *et al.*, *op. cit.* (1998).

[134] 📖 Sicherer and Malloy, *op. cit.*, page 22.

[135] 📖 Hourihane *et al.*, *op. cit.* (1996).

136   Young, *op. cit.*, pages 83-84.

137   P. Vadas *et al.*, "Detection of Peanut Allergens in Breast Milk of Lactating Women," *Journal of the American Medical Association*, Volume 285, 2001, pages 1746-1748.

     Ber, *op. cit.*

     International Agency for Research on Cancer, "Aflatoxins," *Inchem*, Volume 82, 2002, page 171.

138   DiPaolo *et al.*, *op. cit.*

139   European Medicines Agency, "Public Statement on the Allergenic Potency of Herbal Medicinal Products Containing Soya or Peanut Protein," 2006, report EMEA/138139.

     T. Klemola *et al.*, "Feeding a Soy Formula to Children with Cow's Milk Allergy: The Development of Immunoglobulin E-Mediated Allergy to Soy and Peanuts," *Pediatric Allergy and Immunology*, Volume 16, 2005, pages 641-646.

140   See, for example, the Learning Early About Peanut Allergy (LEAP) study, www.leapstudy.co.uk, in progress.

141   P. W. Ewan, "Clinical Study of Peanut and Nut Allergy in 62 Consecutive Patients: New Features and Associations," *British Medical Journal*, Volume 312, 1996, pages 1074-1078.

     R. K. Chandra *et al.*, "Influence of Maternal Diet during Lactation and Use of Formula Feeds on Development of Atopic Eczema in High Risk Infants, *British Medical Journal* Volume 299, 1989, pages 228-230.

     A. S. Kemp, "Allergy Prevention – What We Thought We Knew," *Medical Journal of Australia*, Volume 178, 2003, pages 254-255.

142   Sicherer and Malloy, *op. cit.*, page 158. In this study, half of the mothers transferred protein; concentration was highest about an hour after eating peanuts, and undetectable after four hours in most cases.

143   S. M. Maxwell *et al.*, "Aflatoxin in Breast Milk, Neonatal Cord Blood and Sera of Pregnant Women," *Toxin Reviews*, Volume 8, 1989, pages 19-29.

144   P. G. Holt and C. A. Jones, "The Development of the Immune System During Pregnancy and Early Life," *Allergy*, Volume 55, 2000, pages 688-697.

     National Institute of Allergy and Infectious Diseases, "Immune System Development and the Genesis of Asthma," 2003, funding application AI-03-

041 to the United States National Institutes of Health, *grants.nih.gov/ grants/ guide/ rfa-files/ RFA-AI-03-041.html*.

145 📖 Sicherer and Malloy, *op. cit.*, page 24.

146 📖 A. Holmes-Siedle and L. Adams, *Handbook of Radiation Effects, 2nd edition*, New York: Oxford University Press, 2002.

147 📖 Center for International Earth Science Information Network (CIESIN), *Suppression of the Immune System from Increased Ultraviolet-B Exposure due to Ozone Depletion*, New York: Columbia University, n.d.

148 📖 E. L. Hurwitz and H. Morgenstern, "Effects of Diphtheria-tetanus-pertussis or Tetanus Vaccination on Allergies and Allergy-related Respiratory Symptoms among Children and Adolescents in the United States" *Journal of Manipulative and Physiological Therapeutics*, Volume 23, 2000, pages 81-90.

📖 A. B. Olesen *et al.*, "Atopic Dermatitis Is Increased Following Vaccination for Measles, Mumps and Rubella or Measles Infection," *Acta Dermato-Venereologica*, Volume 83, 2003, pages 445-450.

📖 T. G. Krause *et al.*, "BCG Vaccination and Risk of Atopy," *Journal of the American Medical Association*, Volume 289, 2003, pages 1012-1015.

📖 R. M. D. Bernsen *et al.*, "Lower Rates of Atopic Disorders in Whole Cell Pertussis-Vaccinated Children," *European Respiratory Journal*, Volume 22, 2003, pages 962-964.

149 📖 A. W. Taylor-Robinson, "Multiple Vaccination Effects on Atopy," *Allergy*, Volume 54, 1999, pages 398-400.

150 📖 C. Grüber and K. P. Paul, "Tuberculin Reactivity and Allergy," *Allergy*, Volume 57, 2002, pages 277-280.

📖 H. Hogenesch et al., "Effect of Vaccination on Serum Concentrations of Total and Antigen-Specific Immunoglobulin E in Dogs," *American Journal of Veterinary Research*, Volume 63, 2002, pages 611-616.

151 📖 National Advisory Committee on Immunization, "Supplementary Statement MMR Vaccine and Anaphylactic Hypersensitivity to Egg or Egg-Related Antigens," *Canada Communicable Disease Report*, July 2006.

152 Most scientific authors seem to dispute this entirely; some consider a link to mild skin reactions. See, for example:

📖 A. Patrizi *et al.*, "Sensitization to Thimerosal in Atopic Children," *Contact Dermatitis*, Volume 40, 1999, pages 94-97.

📖 H. Odelram et al., "Immunoglobulin E and G Responses to Pertussis Toxin after Booster Immunization in Relation to Atopy, Local Reactions and Aluminum Content of the Vaccines," *Pediatric Allergy and Immunology*, Volume 5, 1994, pages 118-123.

153 📖 S. Illi et al., "Early Childhood Infectious Diseases and the Development of Asthma up to School Age: A Birth Cohort Study," *British Medical Journal*, Volume 322, 2001, pages 390-395.

154 📖 J. J. Cedra, "Influences of Microbiota on Intestinal Immune System Development," *American Journal of Clinical Nutrition*, Volume 69, 1999, pages 1046S-1051S.

155 📖 A.-L. Ponsonby et al., "Relationship between Early Life Respiratory Illness, Family Size over Time, and the Development of Asthma and Hay Fever: A Seven Year Follow Up Study," *Thorax*, Volume 54, 1999, pages 664-669. Here and in other studies, children with few or zero siblings have been found more likely to have asthma.

156 📖 Lack et al., *op. cit.*

157 📖 L. A. Hanson et al., "Breast Feeding, Infant Formulas, and the Immune System," *Annals of Allergy, Asthma and Immunology*, Volume 90, 2003, pages 59-63.

📖 United States Government Accountability Office, *Breastfeeding*, February 2006, report GAO–06–282.

158 This is different from the difficulty digesting lactose sugar in milk. 📖 A. Host, "Frequency of Cow's Milk Allergy in Childhood," *Annals of Allergy, Asthma and Immunology*, Volume 89, 2002, pages 33-37.

159 💻 Allergy Society of South Africa, "Milk Allergy & Intolerance," www.allergysa.org/milk.htm.

160 📖 H. McGee, *On Food and Cooking*, New York: Scribner, 2004, page 19.

161 📖 Polosa, *op. cit.*

📖 M. Brauer et al., "Air Pollution and the Development of Asthma, Allergies and Infections in a Birth Cohort," *European Respiratory Journal*, 2007, publication pending.

162 📖 M. M. Finkelstein, "Traffic Air Pollution and Mortality Rate Advancement Periods," *American Journal of Epidemiology*, Volume 160, 2004, pages 173-177.

📖 Y. Fuji et al., "Effect of Air Pollution and Environmental Tobacco Smoke on Serum Hyaluronate Concentrations in School Children," *Occupational and Environmental Medicine*, Volume 59, 2002, pages 124-128.

163 📖 S. Romagnani, "Immunologic Influences on Allergy and the TH1/TH2 Balance," *Journal of Allergy and Clinical Immunology*, Volume 113, 2004, pages 395-400.

164 📖 Sicherer and Malloy, *op. cit.*, page 4.

165 For a discussion of how foods affect the liver, see 📖 Pitchford, *op. cit.*, pages 276-290.

166 There is even the case of a non-allergic person who had peanut-specific IgE in their liver, after they received it by transplant from a peanut-allergic person. The same has been found with bone marrow transplant but not kidney transplant. 📖 Young, *op. cit.*, pages 32-33.

📖 C. Legendre et al., "Transfer of Symptomatic Peanut Allergy to the Recipient of a Combined Liver-and-Kidney Transplant," *New England Journal of Medicine*, Volume 338, 1998, pages 202-203.

167 📖 I. Amla et al., "Cirrhosis in Children from Peanut Meal Contaminated by Aflatoxin," *American Journal of Clinical Nutrition*, Volume 24, 1971, pages 609-614.

📖 Cope, *op. cit.*

168 📖 A. Keshavarzian et al., "Leaky Gut in Alcoholic Cirrhosis: A Possible Mechanism for Alcohol-Induced Liver Damage," *American Journal of Gastroenterology*, Volume 94, 1999, pages 200-207.

169 📖 T. Jalonen, "Identical Intestinal Permeability Changes in Children with Different Clinical Manifestations of Cow's Milk Allergy," *Journal of Allergy and Clinical Immunology*, Volume 88, 1991, pages 737-742.

170 📖 D. de Boissieu et al., "Multiple Food Allergy: A Possible Diagnosis in Breastfed Infants," *Acta Pediatrica*, Volume 86, 1997, pages 1042-1046.

171 📖 W. A. Walker, "Pathophysiology of Intestinal Uptake and Absorption of Antigens in Food Allergy," *Annals of Allergy*, Volume 59, 1987, pages 7-16.

📖 Jalonen, *op. cit.*

172 📖 J. M. Kelso et al., "Psychosomatic Peanut Allergy," *Journal of Allergy and Clinical Immunology*, Volume 111, 2003, pages 650-651.

173 These seem better recognized by the psychological literature than by the medical literature.

📖 A. Cziboly et al., "Investigating the Placebo Effect on Food Allergic and Food Aversive Patients," *Magyar Pszichologiai Szemle*, Volume 58, 2003, pages 495-516.

📖 K. Miller, "Psychoneurological Aspects of Food Allergy," *Stress, the Immune System and Psychiatry*, Oxford: Wiley, 1995, pages 185-206.

📖 M. H. Vatn, "Food Intolerance and Psychosomatic Experience," *Scandinavian Journal of Work, Environment and Health*, Volume 23, 1997, pages 75-78.

📖 M. E. Hyland, "The Influence of Beliefs on the Quality of Life of Patients with Allergic Diseases," *Clinical and Experimental Allergy*, Volume 29, 1999, pages 1591-1592.

174 📖 J. J. Walsh, "Influence of Mind on Food Digestion," *Psychotherapy: Including the History of the Use of Mental Influence, Directly and Indirectly in Healing and the Principles for the Application of Energies Derived from the Mind to the Treatment of Disease*, New York: Appleton, 1912, pages 242-249.

175 📖 K. B. Koh and C. S. Hong, "The Relationship of Stress with Serum IgE Level in Patients with Bronchial Asthma," *Yonsei Medical Journal*, Volume 34, 1993, pages 166-174.

📖 M. Timonen, *The Association between Atopic Disorders and Depression: The Northern Finland 1966 Birth Cohort Study*, Oulu: Oulu University, 2003, PhD thesis, section 2.9.1.

The Full Medical

176 Low dose is, for example, a drop in food or on skin; high dose, ingestion of a half peanut or more. In most cases, the dose isn't known at the time, so has to be estimated after the fact.

177 This too is usually estimated after the fact. It may reflect metabolism of the allergen and/or wearing on and off of medication.

178 A local dose – say, initial contact on lips or throat – is one that has not yet had the time to be metabolized.

179 This can be meditating, breathing deep, relaxing, having fun, bringing loved ones close, and so on.

180 Typically, 5 to 30 seeds. Milk thistle is a plant with potent liver cleansing and reinvigorating abilities. 📖 M. Tierra, *Planetary Herbology*, Twin Lakes, WI: Lotus Press, 1988, page 113.

[181] Typically, 1 to 4 pills of 25 mg each.

[182] Typically, 0.3 mL of 0.1% solution.

[183] In terms of the hormonal effect, I'm thinking of cortisone drugs: they mimic the *cortisol* anti-inflammatory released by the adrenal glands, upon a signal from the pituitary gland, under orders from the hypothalamus, in response to perceived stress; used regularly, they can teach this production-and-release loop that it isn't as necessary. 📖 J. R. Hodges and J. Sadow, "Hypothalamo-pituitary-adrenal Function in the Rat after Prolonged Treatment with Cortisol," *British Journal of Pharmacology*, Volume 36, 1969, pages 489-495. 📖 S. J. Lupien *et al.*, "Cortisol Levels During Human Aging Predict Hippocampal Atrophy and Memory Deficits," *Nature Neuroscience*, Volume 1, 1998, pages 69-73.

Epinephrine drugs replace adrenaline in much the same way. If taken regularly, for allergies, there might be an analogous risk. Though here we're talking about occasional anaphylaxis, so that's probably not rational. My habit also comes from once having received the doctor's insert (rather than the patient's one) with my Epipen and read that there's a small chance of heart damage or stroke if taken prematurely, when reaction is absent or mild.

Adrenaline and cortisol are our two most important stress-response agents, and share the same pituitary messenger (*adrenocorticotropic hormone*).

Synthesis

[184] 💻 IMS Health, "Shake-Up for US Antihistamine Market," www.imshealth.com/ web/ content/ 0,3148,64576068_ 63872702_ 70261006_ 70324491,00.html. That share has since declined, as some prescription meds have become available over-the-counter. About $140 million of Benadryl are sold in a year in the US. 📖 "Cold/Allergy/Sinus," *Chain Drug Review*, June 30, 2008, page 173.

[185] 📖 J. Stein, "Art Museum Honoring Rieveschl with Medal," *Cincinnati Post*, November 4, 1999.

The Peanut Detective Bod

[186] See note 50.

[187] 📖 United States Department of Agriculture, *op. cit.* (2002).

[188] 📖 P. J. D'Adamo, *Live Right for Your Type*, New York: Putnam, 2001, pages 195-219.

[189] Meridians are energy pathways, in traditional Chinese medicine. Each one has a specific path through the head torso, and/or limbs, and is associated with certain organs and functions.

[190] Chemically speaking, lemon juice is strongly acidic. In traditional Chinese medicine, it is acidic outside the body but alkalizing inside.

My Game Plan

[191] See note 22.

[192] Enzymes are proteins that speed up *(catalyze)* the breakdown of food. Each part of the digestive tract has some. For example, there are amylases to turn starch to sugars, lipases to turn fat to fatty acids, and proteases and peptidases to turn protein to amino acids. Enzymes can be destroyed by prolonged or high heat during storage, cooking, preserving, refining, and sterilization *(pasteurization)*.

My approach has to do with the difference between "healthy" and "clean." For example, I don't generally soap-wash or peel my vegetables. From what I've studied and felt, most don't have much pesticide to begin with, washing doesn't make much of a difference, and peeling doesn't get it all either, whereas it does eliminate important nutrients, make food go stale faster, take time and effort, and create waste; it may also reduce immunity built by moderate exposure to microbes.

"Healthy" implies that food be grown in soil kept fertile by crop rotation, amendment with compost, and other practices. It does not necessarily mean "organic:" often, compared to non-organic produce, certified organic goods are more expensive, have traveled further/longer, fill me up no more, and feel or taste worse. Healthy also doesn't necessarily mean vegetarian, especially when meat is replaced with large amounts or complex combinations of rich foods (like dairy, eggs, soy, or nuts, many of which also happen to be grown relatively intensively).

[193] I don't like the quality of city tap water, don't find carbon-filtration much of an improvement, and find bottled water worse and more expensive. Letting tap water stand seems to get rid of some of the unpleasant and harsh chlorine used to sterilize it. Reverse-osmosis filtered water feels good, but still missing something: life, minerals, and softness. Putting a piece of dry kelp seaweed in my bottle seems to bring it back.

The idea came from a search for a way to slowly, deeply nourish my joints. I'd been having knee and hip problems, and was concerned I might be on the family path to arthritis. I'd heard of using animal parts to heal the same parts of ourselves, but there was only so much ligament and tendon I wanted to eat! Plant mucilage felt like an equivalent. It's abundant in marshmallow root, flax seed, kelp, and some other foods. Whole kelp is the one that felt and tasted best. My joints have improved a lot since, whether for this reason or others.

194   In a way, this is about handling positive stress. Again, the idea is to sustain keen feeling without blowing out. It can amount to anything from savouring a meal to drawing out an orgasm or going for a thorough work-out.

195   Fermentation uses bacteria, molds, or other microorganisms to predigest a food and change its properties. The goal may be to make it more digestible, preserve it, leaven it, improve its taste, and/or something else. Fermentation often makes a food more alkaline. Some examples are miso, soy sauce, yogurt, sauerkraut, and sourdough bread.

There are other traditions of fermenting legumes, such as 📖 O. K. Achi, "Traditional Fermented Protein Condiments in Nigeria," *African Journal of Biotechnology*, Volume 4, 2005, pages 1612-1621.

196   See note 190.

197   Likewise, if a skin test or RAST showed that I had a high peanut-specific IgE count, that would make it more likely I'm still strongly allergic and shouldn't experiment. 📖 Sicherer and Malloy, *op. cit.*, page 81.

198   There are different ways to make sprouts. I soak the peanuts (or other seeds) overnight, in a bowl, then drain and rinse them twice a day. The sprout usually appears after 2-4 days; after a few more days, roots and leaves appear. I've eaten them at every stage, and prefer those from early in the sprouting process.

Fermenting the nuts would be another option. It hasn't appealed to me as much, based on experience with fermented soy, or seemed to bring the same quality of energy as sprouting.

199   While this has been going on, I've been doing some other reprogramming: learning to be ambidextrous.

I grew up left-handed (*sinister*) at some things, like writing, and right-handed (*dextrous*) at others, like throwing. I held my pen/pencil a "wrong" way and was said to have hand-eye coordination trouble. Over time, I found I could do some things, like racquet sports, decently on either side (*ambidextrously*, literally meaning "with two right hands"). It hasn't always been the best way to advance fast, and in a way that's the point: I already felt I was moving too fast and under too much pressure. It's fun, and brings resilience.

The Sprouted Peanut Vaccine and Other Stories

For example, when I develop a chronic pain or impairment because of repetitive stress (doing the same task the same way, over and over, and fast), switching hands can help in many ways. It stops stressing one limb, while letting me get the job done with the other one; at first this slows my work and reduces its quality, but that saves the stress of perfectionism, and things still tend to get done well enough and on time. Sometimes my second side figures out a more efficient way of doing things; then my first side can learn it, and this can fix whatever overcompensation was causing the repetitive stress in the first place. Or I can carry on with two different ways of doing the task, in other words with more creativity: for example, when I started drawing with my right hand I found I could express my vision better.

My second side can teach me about how I learn, since my first side chose its habits before I can remember, sometimes under pressure. This gives me an action-based picture of the reprogramming I've done inside to handle peanut allergy and other problems. Some of the findings and methods may be useful to other people, as-is or for what they say about human capacity.

200 Sicherer and Malloy, *op. cit.*, pages 47-77. Young, *op. cit.*, pages 6-14 and 23-24.

201 See note 30.

202 See notes 135, 136, and 139.

Related Symptoms

203 Restore Unity, "Natural Method – Antihistamine," *www.restoreunity.org/ natural_method_antihistamine.htm*.

204 K.-G. Wenzel, "Dr. Med. K.-G. Wenzel," *www.dr-wenzel-limburg.de*.

205 A. W. Saul, "Orthomolecular Medicine Hall of Fame," *orthomolecular.org/ hof/ index.shtml*.

206 National Academy of Sciences, "Biographical Memoirs: Linus Carl Pauling," *www.nap.edu/ html/ biomems/ lpauling.html*.

Wikipedia, "Linus Pauling," *en.wikipedia.org/ wiki/ Linus_Pauling*.

207 L. Pauling, "Modern Structural Chemistry," *Nobel Lectures, Chemistry, 1942-1962*, Amsterdam: Elsevier, 1964, pages 429-427.

L. Pauling, "Science and Peace," *Nobel Lectures, Peace, 1951-1970*, Amsterdam: Elsevier, 1972, pages 271-287.

208 "Nambudripad's Allergy Elimination Techniques," *www.naet.com*.

209 📖 Cutler, *op. cit.*, pages 299-303. 💻 "BioSET," *www.bioset.net*.

Related Systems

210 📖 A. Morrier, *Shiatsu: Formation de base*, Montreal: Centre de santé intégrale Guijek, 2004, page 28. 📖 Pitchford, *op. cit.*, page 265.

Unchosen Experiments

211 The whole quote goes, "No man is an Island, entire of itself; every man is a piece of the Continent, a part of the main; if a clod be washed away by the sea, Europe is the less, as well as if a promontory were, as well as if a manor of thy friends or of thine own were; any man's death diminishes me, because I am involved in Mankind; And therefore never send to know for whom the bell tolls; It tolls for thee." 📖 John Donne, *Meditation XVII*, 17th century, copyright expired.

The Biology of Stress and Pleasure

212 📖 E. C. Marieb, *Human Anatomy and Physiology*, Redwood City, CA: Benjamin-Cummings, 1995.

213 Since phenylalanine is the precursor of the tanning pigment melanin, these people tend to be blond and light-skinned.

📖 R. L. Trites and H. Tryphonas, "Food Intolerance and Hyperactivity," *Topics in Early Childhood Special Education*, Volume 3, 1983, pages 49-54.

📖 F. Feillet, "Phenylketonuria," *Presse Médicale*, Volume 35, 2006, pages 502-508.

💻 Mayo Clinic, "Phenylketonuria" *www.mayoclinic.com/ health/ phenylketonuria/ DS00514/ DSECTION=2.*

214 📖 Cutler, *op cit.*, pages 70-71.

215 Heavy, regular use of some of these ultimately depresses serotonin.

📖 B. G. Katzung, *op. cit.*

📖 E. Tal *et al.*, "Effect of Air Ionization on Blood Serotonin *In Vitro*," *Cellular and Molecular Life Sciences*, Volume 32, 1976, pages 326-327.

Blood Type, Body Type, Feels Good

216   📖 D'Adamo, *op. cit.*, pages 1-15.

217   📖 D'Adamo, *op. cit.*, pages 1-15.

218   For example, when the US population is divided along lines that are part-ethnic and part-skin-colour: Natives are mostly (79%) O, with almost no AB; whites, mostly O (45%) and B (40%); blacks, mostly O (49%), B (27%), and A (20%); and Asians, mostly O (40%), B (28%), and A (27%). 📖 E. C. Marieb, *Human Anatomy and Physiology*, Redwood City, CA: Benjamin-Cummings, 2004, page 630.

219   📖 D'Adamo, *op. cit.*, pages 195-219.

220   See note 53.

221   For each type, there are people who secrete antigens into body fluids and people who don't. The recommendations for secretors and non-secretors are different for some foods.

222   📖 Frawley, *op. cit.*, pages 83-94.

Cancer

223   📖 M. Gerson, *A Cancer Therapy: Results of Fifty Cases & The Cure of Advanced Cancer by Diet Therapy*, San Diego: The Gerson Institute, 2002, pages 22-28, 35-36, 135-138, and 187-191.

224   In particular, Gerson was concerned with the balance between sodium and potassium. The former should dominate in *anodic* fluids and tissues (blood serum, lymph, tendons, ligaments, thyroid, bile ducts, and so on), representing 30% of the body; the latter, in *cathodic* tissues (muscles, heart, liver, kidney cortex, brain, and so on), representing 60% of the body; with 10% of the body being neither exactly one nor the other. Each has its own set of vitamins and enzymes, and the two have opposite electrical natures. In normal functioning, sodium, chloride, and water enter the potassium tissues during the day and are eliminated in morning urine. Excess dietary sodium, however, leads to mineral and fluid retention in the potassium tissues, followed by infection, poisoning, and leakage of potassium (and glycogen), which in turn worsens the body's imbalance.

225   📖 M. Kushi and A. Jack, *The Cancer Prevention Diet*, Wellingborough, UK: Thorsons, 1984, pages 3-50, 63-77, 98-107, and 118.

226   See note 83 about nightshade and onion family plants. Cabbages are kin to broccoli, cauliflower, brussels sprouts, kale, mustard, turnips, radishes, and more.

Wild Speculation

227 The idea of a "last line of defense" is explored, for example, in 📖 M. Profet, "The Function of Allergy: Immunological Defense against Toxins," *Quarterly Review of Biology*, Volume 66, 1991, pages 23-62.

228 📖 *The Top 10 Causes of Death*, Geneva: World Health Organization, 2007, fact sheet 310.

229 💻 United States Centers for Disease Control and Prevention, "Leading Causes of Death, 1900 to 1998," *www.cdc.gov/ nchs/ data/ dvs/ lead1900_98.pdf*.

230 For example, the first National Cancer Survey was only done in 1937.

231 📖 S. Peters, *The Land in Trust: A Social History of the Organic Farming Movement*, Montreal: McGill University, 1979, pages 70-74, PhD thesis.

📖 A. Davidson, ed., *The Oxford Companion to Food*, Oxford, UK: Oxford University Press, 1999, page 855.

📖 J. Birch et al., eds., *Larousse Gastronomique*, New York: Clarkson Potter, 2001, page 155.

232 📖 W. A. Price, *Nutrition and Physical Degeneration*, La Mesa, CA: Price–Pottenger Nutrition Foundation, 2000. The book is also available online at *gutenberg.net.au/ ebooks02/ 0200251h.html*.

Price went among the following peoples: Inuit and various aboriginals of Canada and the US, various aboriginals of Peru, Scottish islanders, alpine Swiss, various tribes of central and eastern Africa, and various aboriginals of Australia, New Zealand and the South Pacific.

233 📖 C. Davis and E. Saltos, "Dietary Recommendations and How They Have Changed Over Time," Washington: United States Department of Agriculture report AIB–750, 1999, pages 33–50.

📖 Pitchford, *op. cit.* looks at what various cultures have eaten over time – whole grains, legumes, fish, meat, dairy, vegetables, fruit, and so on – and how this relates to health and environmental sustainability. For example, the protein idea is challenged because it may come from a misinterpretation of old studies on lab rats, and because heavy meat-eating can imply deforestation, animal abuse, or colon cancer.

234 📖 M. Harris, *Our Kind: Who We Are, Where We Came From, Where We Are Going*, New York: Harper Perennial, 1989, pages 166-168.

235 📖 N. I. Vavilov, *Origin and Geography of Cultivated Plants*, Cambridge: Cambridge University Press, 1992.

236 Though it's hard to know for sure, health and environment seem to be consistently among the top priorities of people in the First World. See, for example:

💻 "Environment a Priority for More Canadians, Poll Suggests," *CBC News*, November 8, 2006, www.cbc.ca/ canada/ story/ 2006/ 11/ 08/ environment-poll.html.

💻 "Americans Want to Spend More on Education, Health," University of Chicago National Opinion Research Center, January 10, 2007, www-news.uchicago.edu/ releases/ 07/ 070110. gss. shtml.

💻 "'Health Should Be Top Priority'," *BBC News*, April 15, 2007, news.bbc.co.uk/ 1/ hi/ health/ 6549709.stm.

💻 "Les services publics trouvent grâce aux yeux des Français," *TF1*, June 18, 2007, tf1.lci.fr/ infos/ economie/ consommation/ 0,,3471972,00-services-publics-trouvent-grace-aux-yeux-francais-.html.

💻 M. Shroff, "Announcing the 2006 UMR Survey of Public Opinion: A Chance to Hear What Consumers Say about Privacy in Business," New Zealand Privacy Commissioner, March 30, 2006, www.privacy.org.nz/ library/ announcing-the-2006-umr-survey-of-public-opinion-a-chance-to-hear-what-consumers-say-about-privacy-in-business-marie-shroff.

237 📖 Cutler, *op. cit.*, pages 127-128.

238 💻 G6PD Deficiency Association, "What is G6PD Deficiency," Venice: Associazione Italiana Favismo – Deficit di G6PD, www.g6pd.org/ favism/ english/ index.mv?pgid=intro.

📖 E. Sartori, "On the Pathogenesis of Favism," *Journal of Medical Genetics*, Volume 8, 1971, pages 462-467.

239 💻 P. Wong, "Gilbert's Syndrome: A Patient's Guide," www.medic8.com/ healthguide/ articles/ gilbertsyn.html.

📖 M. D. Cappellini *et al.* "The Interaction between Gilbert's Syndrome and G6PD Deficiency Influences Bilirubin Levels," *British Journal of Haematology*, Volume 104, 1999, pages 928-929.

240 📖 E. M. del Giudice *et al.*, "Coinheritance of Gilbert Syndrome Increases the Risk for Developing Gallstones in Patients With Hereditary Spherocytosis," *Blood*, Volume 94, 1999, pages 2259-2262.

241 For example, Canada's 2001 Census of Agriculture gives the following livestock population data. Cattle: 2% bulls, 38% cows, 16% heifers 1 year and over, 11% steers 1 year and over, 33% calves. Sheep: 2% rams, 50% ewes, 48%

lambs. Pigs: 0.3% boars, 10% sows and gilts for breeding, 34% nursing and weaner pigs, 56% grower and finishing pigs. 📖 *www.statcan.ca/ english/ freepub/ 95F0301XIE/ tables.htm.*

242 See, for example, 📖 C. V. Bagley, "Acute and Subacute Ruminal Acidosis," Utah State University Extension Service, *extension.usu.edu/ files/ publications/ newsletter/ pub__5621800.html.*

243 📖 R. Manning, "The Oil We Eat," *Harper's Magazine,* February 2004, pages 37-45.

244 🎧 C. Barnes, interview by A. Gottlieb, "Corn, Beans, Squash, and Survival," *Native Solidarity News,* Episode 340, 2003, first broadcast on CKUT 90.3 FM Radio McGill. Barnes had been raising and sharing traditional varieties of corn for 50 years, and come to the program via the Native American Diabetes Project.

Also, see 📖 Y. I. Kwon *et al.,* "Health Benefits of Traditional Corn, Beans, and Pumpkin: In Vitro Studies for Hyperglycemia and Hypertension Management," *Journal of Medicinal Food,* Volume 10, 2007, pages 266-275.

Reforming Animal Nature

245 📖 J. Diamond. *Guns, Germs, and Steel: The Fates of Human Societies,* New York: Norton, 1999, pages 159 and 169-174.

Some Things Don't Make Sense

246 📖 J. Khan, "Un rapport canadien appelle à négocier avec les talibans," *La Presse,* March 2, 2007, page A17, photo by S. Marai of Agence France-Presse.

Conclusion

247 For example, Julius Wagner-Jauregg found that the dementia associated with advanced syphilis could be reversed by deliberately infecting patients with malaria. For this he earned the 1927 Nobel Prize in Medicine. 📖 J. Wagner-Jauregg, "The Treatment of Dementia Paralytica by Malaria Inoculation," *Nobel Lectures, Physiology or Medicine, 1922-1941,* Amsterdam: Elsevier, 1965, pages 159-172.

Also see note 153 about how some early-childhood infection, or multiple infection in general, may prevent asthma.

The Sprouted Peanut Vaccine and Other Stories

Selected Bibliography

E. Cutler, *The Food Allergy Cure*, New York: Three Rivers Press, 2003.

P. J. D'Adamo, *Live Right for Your Type*, New York: Putnam, 2001.

A. Davidson, ed., *The Oxford Companion to Food*, Oxford, UK: Oxford University Press, 1999.

J. Diamond. *Guns, Germs, and Steel: The Fates of Human Societies*, New York: Norton, 1999.

D. Frawley, *Ayurvedic Healing*, Twin Lakes, WI: Lotus Press, 2000.

M. Harris, *Our Kind: Who We Are, Where We Came From, Where We Are Going*, New York: Harper Perennial, 1989.

M. Jackson, *Allergy: The History of a Modern Malady*, London: Reaktion, 2006.

B. Katzung, ed., *Basic and Clinical Pharmacology*, New York: McGraw-Hill, 2003.

C. D. Klaassen *et al.*, eds., *Casarett and Doull's Toxicology*, New York: McGraw-Hill, 1991, pages 565-622.

M. Kushi and A. Jack, *The Cancer Prevention Diet*, Wellingborough, UK: Thorsons, 1984.

R. Maiti, ed., *The Peanut (Arachis Hypogaea) Crop*, Enfield, NH: Science Publishers, 2002.

E. C. Marieb, *Human Anatomy and Physiology*, Redwood City, CA: Benjamin-Cummings, 1995.

D. Nambudripad, *NAET: Say Good-Bye to Your Allergies*, Buena Park, CA: Delta Publishing, 2003.

P. Pitchford, *Healing with Whole Foods*, Berkeley: North Atlantic Books, 1993.

W. A. Price, *Nutrition and Physical Degeneration*, La Mesa, CA: Price–Pottenger Nutrition Foundation, 2000.

S. H. Sicherer and T. Malloy, *The Complete Peanut Allergy Handbook*, New York: Berkley Books, 2005.

A. F. Smith, *Peanuts: The Illustrious History of the Goober Pea*, Chicago: University of Illinois Press, 2002.

M. Spraycar, ed., *Stedman's Medical Dictionary*, Baltimore: Williams and Wilkins, 1995.

L. M. Tierney Jr. et al., eds., *Current Medical Diagnosis and Treatment*, New York: Lange, 2006.

M. Tierra, *Planetary Herbology*, Twin Lakes, WI: Lotus Press, 1988.

N. I. Vavilov, *Origin and Geography of Cultivated Plants*, Cambridge: Cambridge University Press, 1992.

M. C. Young, *The Peanut Allergy Answer Book*, Gloucester, MA: Fair Winds Press, 2001.

Allergy

American Journal of Clinical Nutrition

Annals of Allergy, Asthma, and Immunology

British Medical Journal

Clinical and Experimental Allergy

Current Allergy and Asthma Reports

Current Opinion in Allergy and Clinical Immunology

Journal of Allergy and Clinical Immunology

Journal of Immunology

Journal of the American Medical Association

New England Journal of Medicine

Pediatric Allergy and Immunology

Thorax

International and National Allergy Organizations

This listing is up-to-date as of Fall 2008. As far as I know, these are all non-profits. Most are linked to the World Allergy Organization website, included below, so new contact information can be checked there. Phone and fax country codes are given in brackets. The only state or provincial organizations included are those that serve a linguistic minority.

There are many private websites on food allergy, such as allallergy.net, allergicchild.com, allergicliving.com, beyondapeanut.com, foodallergytalk.com, food-allergens.de, kidswithfoodallergies.org, mdlinx.com/allergyimmunolinx, peanutallergy.com, and peanutaware.com.

This listing is meant to be complete, and implies neither endorsement of an organization nor verification of its public information.

International

Australasian Society of Clinical Immunology and Allergy
PO Box 450 Balgowlah NSW 2093, Australia
Fax (61) 2 9907 9773
education@allergy.org.au
www.allergy.org.au

European Academy of Allergology and Clinical Immunology
PO Box 24140
S-10451 Stockholm, Sweden
Phone (46) 8 459 6623
Fax (46) 8 663 3815
executive.office@eaaci.org
www.eaaci.net

European Centre for Allergy Research Foundation
Klinik für Dermatologie, Venerologie und Allergologie
Charité - Universitätsmedizin Berlin
Charitéplatz 1
10117 Berlin, Germany
Phone (49) 30 450 518 044
Fax (49) 30 450 518 938
ecarf@charite.de
www.ecarf.org

European Federation of Allergy and Airway Diseases Patients
   Association
35 rue du Congrès
1000 Brussels, Belgium
Phone (32) 2 227 2712
Fax (32) 2 218 3141
info@efanet.org
www.efanet.org

Global Allergy and Asthma European Network
Berlin, Germany
Phone (49) 304 5051 8038
office@ga2len.net
www.ga2len.net

Sociedad Latinomericana de Alergia, Asma e Inmunología
www.slaai.org

UCB Institute of Allergy
3 George Street
Watford, Hertfordshire, WD1 8UH, United Kingdom
Phone (44) 1923 211 811
Fax (44) 1923 229 002
instituteofallergy@ucb-group.com
www.theucbinstituteofallergy.com

World Allergy Organization
Secretariat
555 East Wells Street, Suite 1100
Milwaukee, WI 53202-3823 USA
Phone (1) 414 276 1791
Fax (1) 414 276 3349
info@worldallergy.org
www.worldallergy.org

Albania

Albanian Association in Support of Asthma and Allergy Patients
Rr. Anastas Kullorioti Nr. 8/1
Tirana
Phone (355) 42 69200
Fax (355) 42 69200

Argentina

Asociación Argentina de Alergia e Inmunología Clínica
Moreno 909 - Capital Federal
Buenos Aires
Phone (54) 11 4334 7680
www.alergia.org.ar

Sociedad Argentina de Alergia e Inmunopatalogía
info@saaei.com.ar
www.saaei.com.ar

Australia

Anaphylaxis Australia
PO Box 3182
Asquith NSW 2077
Phone (61) 2 9482 5988

coordinator@allergyfacts.org.au
www.allergyfacts.org.au

Belgium

Fondation pour la prévention des allergies
56 rue de la Concorde
1050 Brussels
Phone (32) 2 511 6761
Fax (32) 2 511 6761
fpa@oasis-allergies.org
www.oasis-allergies.org

Brazil

Associação Brasileira de Alergia e Imunopatologia
Av. Prof. Ascendino Reis, 455 - Vila Clementino
CEP 04027-000
São Paulo, SP
Phone (55) 11 75 6888
Fax (55) 11 72 4069
sbai@sbai.org.br
www.sbai.org.br

Canada

Allergy / Asthma Information Association
111 Zenway Boulevard, Unit 1
Vaughan, Ontario L4H 3H9
Phone (1) 905 265 3322
Fax (1) 905 850 2070
admin@aaia.ca
aaia.ca

Anaphylaxis Canada
2005 Sheppard Avenue East, Suite 800
Toronto, Ontario M2J 5B4
Phone (1) 416 785 5666
Fax (1) 416 785 0458
info@anaphylaxis.ca
www.anaphylaxis.ca

Association québécoise des allergies alimentaires
445, boulevard Sainte-Foy, bureau 100
Longueuil, Québec J4J 1X9
Phone (1) 514 990 2575
Fax (1) 514 990 2575
aqaa@aqaa.qc.ca
www.aqaa.qc.ca

Canadian Allergy, Asthma and Immunology Foundation
774 Echo Drive
Ottawa, Ontario K1S 5N8
Phone (1) 613 730 6272
Fax (1) 613 730 1116
caaid@rcpsc.edu
www.allergyfoundation.ca

Canadian Society of Allergy and Clinical Immunology
774 Echo Drive
Ottawa, Ontario K1S 5N8
Phone (1) 613 730 6272
Fax (1) 613 730 1116
csaci@rcpsc.edu
www.csaci.medical.org

Denmark

Dansk Selskab for Allergologi
Rigshospitalet Allergiklinikken, afs. 4222
Blegdamsvej 9
2100 København
Phone (45) 35 45 75 89
Fax (45) 35 45 75 83
www.danskallergi.dk

Finland

Allergia- ja Astmaliitto ry
Paciuksenkatu 19
00270 Helsinki
Phone (358) 9 473 351
Fax (358) 9 4733 5330
www.allergia.com

France

Société française d'allergologie et d'immunologie clinique
www.sfaic.com

Germany

Deutsche Gesellschaft für Allergologie und Klinische Immunologie
Postfach 700464
81304 München
Phone (49) 89 5466 2968
Fax (49) 89 5838 24
dgaki@t-online.de
www.dgaki.de

Japan

Japan Allergy Foundation
4-5-1 Kudan Minami Chiyodaku
Tokyo
Phone (81) 3 3222 3437
Fax (81) 3 3222 3438

Japanese Society of Allergology
7th Fl., Ishimizu Building
1-35-26 Hongo, Bunkyo-ku
Tokyo 113-0033
Phone (81) 3 3816 0280
Fax (81) 3 3816 0219
info@jsaweb.jp
www.jsaweb.jp

Japanese Society for Immunology
1st Floor, Harashima-Misaki-cho Building
3-6-2 Misaki-cho, Chiyoda-ku
Tokyo 101-0061
Phone (81) 3 3511 9795
Fax (81) 3 3511 9788
www.socnii.ac.jp/jsi2

Malaysia

Malaysian Society of Allergy and Immunology
142 Jalan Ipoh
51200 Kuala Lumpur
Phone (60) 3 4041 6336
Fax (60) 3 4042 6970
www.allergymsai.org

Mexico

Colegio Mexicano de Pediatras Especialistas en Inmunología Clínica y Alergia
Montecito 38-piso 25, Oficina 34
Col. Nápoles, México, D.F. 03810
Phone (52) 55 9000 2008
Fax (52) 55 9000 2008
comaaipe@wtcmexico.com.mx
www.compedia.org.mx

New Zealand

Allergy New Zealand
PO Box 56117, Dominion Road
Auckland
Phone (64) 9 623 3912
Fax (64) 9 623 0091
www.allergy.org.nz

Norway

Nordsk Forening for Allergologi og Immunopatologi
www.legeforeningen.no/index.gan?id=57992&subid=0

Norges Astma- og Allergiforbund
Postboks 2603 St. Hanshaugen
0131 Oslo
Phone (47) 23 35 35 35
Fax (47) 23 35 35 30
naaf@naaf.no
www.naaf.no

Poland

Witamy w Serwisie Alergolicznym
Ośrodek Badonia Alergenów Środowiskowych w Warszawie
Phone (48) 22 865 4200
Fax (48) 22 865 4202
obaswaw@alergen.net
www.alergen.info.pl

Portugal

Sociedade Portuguesa de Alergologia e Imunologia Clínica
Rua Manuel Rodrigues da Silva, 7C - Escritório 1
Telheiras, 1600-503 Lisboa
Phone (351) 217152426
Fax (351) 217152428
spaic@sapo.pt
www.spaic.pt

South Africa

Allergy Society of South Africa
PO Box 88, Observatory 7935
Cape Town
Phone (27) 21 447 9019
Fax (27) 21 448 0846
www.allergysa.org

Spain

Socieded Espanola de Alergología e Immunología Clínica
Secretaría Técnica
Apartado Correos 7029
08080 Barcelona
Phone (34) 93 394 53 69

Fax (34) 93 332 95 60
seaic@seaic.es
www.seaic.es

Societat Catalana d'Allèrgia i Immunologia Clínica
Apartat de Correus 7029
08080 Barcelona
scaic@scaic.cat
www.scaic.cat

Sweden

Svenska föreningen för Allergologi
www.sffa.nu

Switzerland

Swiss Center for Allergy, Skin, and Asthma
Scheibenstrasse 20
3014 Bern
Phone (41) 31 359 90 00
Fax (41) 31 359 90 90
info@ahaswiss.ch
www.ahaswiss.ch

The Netherlands

Nederlands Anafylaxis Netwerk
Oranjelaan 91
3311 DJ Dordrecht
Phone (31) 78 639 03 56
Fax (31) 78 639 02 43
info@anafylaxis.nl
www.anafylaxis.nl

Nederlandse Vereniging voor Allergologie
p/a Erasmus MC sector Allergologie, kamer GK-324
Postbus 2040
3000 CA Rotterdam
secretariaat@nvva-allergologie.nl
www.nvva-allergologie.nl

Turkey

Türkiye Ulusal Allerji ve Klinik İmmünologi Derneği
Hacettepe Üniversitesi Tıp Fakültesi
Çocuk Allerji ve Astma Ünitesi
Hacettepe, 06100, Ankara
Phone (90) 312 324 2511
Fax (90) 312 311 2357
allergy@hacettepe.edu.tr
www.aid.org.tr

United Kingdom

Allergy and Allergies Agency
144 Harley St.
London W1
Phone (44) 1276 510 648
www.allergy-network.co.uk

Allergy UK
3 White Oak Square
London Road
Swanley, Kent BR8 7AG
Phone (44) 1322 619 898
Fax (44) 1322 663 480
info@allergyuk.org
www.allergyuk.org

Anaphylaxis Campaign
PO Box 275
Farnborough GU14 6SX
Phone (44) 1252 546 100
Fax (44) 1252 377 140
info@anaphylaxis.org.uk
www.anaphylaxis.org.uk

British Society for Asthma and Clinical Immunology
17 Doughty Street
London WC1N 2PL
Phone (44) 2074 040 278
Fax (44) 2074 040 280
info@bsaci.org
www.bsaci.org

United States

Allergy and Asthma Network Mothers of Asthmatics
2751 Prosperity Avenue, Suite 150
Fairfax, VA 22031
Phone (1) 703 641 9595
Fax (1) 703 573 7794
www.aanma.org

American Academy of Allergy, Asthma & Immunology
555 East Wells Street, Suite 1100
Milwaukee, WI 53202-3823
Phone (1) 414 272 6071
info@aaaai.org
www.aaaai.org

American Association of Immunologists
9650 Rockville Pike
Bethesda, MD 20814

Phone (1) 301 634 7178
Fax (1) 301 634 7887
infoaai@aai.org
www.aai.org

American College of Allergy, Asthma & Immunology
85 West Algonquin Road, Suite 550
Arlington Heights, IL 60005
Phone (1) 847 4271200
Fax (1) 847 4271294
mail@acaai.org
www.acaai.org

Asthma and Allergy Foundation of America
1233 20th Street Northwest, Suite 402
Washington, DC 20036
Phone (1) 202 727 8462
info@aafa.org
www.aafa.org

Federation of Clinical Immunology Societies
11950 West Lake Park Drive, Suite 320
Milwaukee, WI 53224
Phone (1) 414 359 1670
Fax (1) 414 359 1671
www.focisnet.org

Food Allergy & Anaphylaxis Network
11781 Lee Jackson Highway, Suite 160
Fairfax, VA 22033-3309
Phone (1) 800 929 4040
Fax (1) 703 691 2713
faan@foodallergy.org
www.foodallergy.org

Food Allergy Initiative
1414, Avenue of the Americas, Suite 1804
New York, NY 10019
Phone (1) 212 207 1974
Fax (1) 917 338 5130
info@foodallergyinitiative.org
www.foodallergyinitiative.org

Joint Council of Allergy, Asthma, and Immunology
50 North Brockway, 3-3
Palatine, IL 60067
Phone (1) 847 934 1918
info@jcaai.org
www.jcaai.org

Mayo Clinic Allergy Center
4500 San Pablo Road South
Jacksonville, FL 32224
Phone (1) 904 953 2000
www.mayoclinic.com/health/allergy/aa99999

National Institute of Allergy and Infectious Diseases
Office of Communications and Government Relations
6610 Rockledge Drive, MSC 6612
Bethesda, MD 20892-6612
Phone (1) 301 496 5717
Fax (1) 301 402 3573
www3.niaid.nih.gov

Glossary

Adrenaline. Hormone made by the adrenal glands and released into the bloodstream, under stressful conditions, upon signal from the pituitary gland, in turn triggered by the hypothalamus. Speeds heart rate, dilates pupils, constricts some blood vessels (to retain heat) while dilating others, dilates respiratory vessels, speeds carbohydrate and fat metabolism (to give energy), and relaxes smooth muscle in bronchioles and intestines. This leads to higher blood pressure, bowel action, euphoria, and other effects. Active ingredient in Epipen medicine used to treat anaphylaxis; usually obtained from animals. Also called epinephrine.

Aflatoxin. Toxic mold from the *aspergillus* family. Found in legumes, grains, nuts, milk, and some other foods, as well as in cigarette smoke, household mold, and other substances.

Allergy. Mild or strong, systemic, immune-related, non-life-threatening response to a physically or biochemically active substance that is harmless to most people. May require prior exposure (*sensitization*). For example: swelling of lymph nodes minutes after eating a certain food.

Alpha amino acid. Building block used to make protein. There are about 20, including 10 that we can make aplenty and 10 "essential" ones we must get wholly or partly from food.

Anaphylaxis. Allergy that develops rapidly and intensely enough to cross a threshold of systemic and emotional panic. Can be life-threatening. For example: suffocating after eating or thinking of eating a certain food.

Antigen. Substance that elicits an immune response, including the production of antibodies with which the antigen can combine, upon future exposure.

Arachidonic acid. Polyunsaturated fatty acid made in the body, usually from linoleic acid. Present in most tissues and foods, especially meat, eggs, dairy, shellfish, peanuts, and nori seaweed.

Source of inflammatory leukotrienes, prostaglandin, and thromboxanes. Important for central nervous system functioning.

Asthma. Moderate or severe, ongoing or episodic breathing trouble, due to swelling and/or mucus in the airways (lungs, bronchi, trachea, pharynx, and/or nose) plus spasming of the muscles around them. There is a baseline condition of vulnerability, such that when an allergen (such as cigarette smoke or animal secretions) is inhaled, histamine and other inflamers are released. May also be cause or worsened by stress, strenuous exercise, colds, and so on.

Autism. Pattern of mental and social development problems such as impaired communication, physical awkwardness, narrow focus, social withdrawal, and behaviour "loops." Results from genetic damage done by a toxic substance or another factor.

Ayurveda. East Indian medical tradition using foods, herbs, massage, and more. Includes a system of understanding body, feelings, and outside influences in terms of air (*vata*), water (*kapha*), and fire (*pitta*) elements.

Calorie. Unit of energy. One calorie is what it takes to heat up, or what is recovered from cooling down, 1 gram of water by 1 degree Celsius. The nutritional "calorie" is a kilocalorie, equal to 1000 calories.

Cancer. Runaway and often faulty reproduction of cells. This can strain healthy tissues and make masses (*tumours*) of useless tissue that, in turn, can invade surrounding areas, spread (*metastasize*) far across the body, and/or regrow after being cut out. In contrast, *non-malignant* tumours don't spread. Often fatal, especially if untreated. Can be due to a genetic glitch caused by a pollutant, disease, stress, and so on.

Carbohydrate. Foodstuff made of carbon, hydrogen, and oxygen. Includes sugars, starches, glycogen, cellulose, chitin, and other substances used for energy, structure, and more. Also called *saccharide*.

Carcinogenic. Regularly found to cause cancer.

Depression. Literally, a drop or low-point. "Clinical" depression refers to an ongoing bad emotional feeling that makes it hard to function: maintain body processes, do work, socialize, and so on.

Diphenhydramine. Non-prescription anti-histamine, also known as Benadryl. Works by preventing cells, in the respiratory tract and elsewhere, from absorbing inflammatory histamine released into the blood following exposure to an allergen.

Eczema. Skin condition that tends to progress from tiny blisters to reddening, itching, swelling, emitting fluid, crusting, and flaking.

Enzyme. Catalyst of a biological process, such as food digestion. Different types are found throughout the digestive tract. For example, there are amylases to turn carbohydrates to sugars, proteases and peptidases to turn proteins to amino acids, and lipases to turn fats to fatty acids.

Fat. Substance made from carbon, hydrogen, and oxygen, with a typical structure of chains (*fatty acids*) attached to a spine of glycerol. The chain length and the position and number of reactive (*unsaturated*) carbon-carbon bonds affects how the fat behaves in and out of the body: solid or liquid, stable or able to go rancid, easy or hard to digest, and so on. Also called *lipid*.

Histamine. Inflammatory substance made from histidine, an amino acid especially abundant in some meats, dairy, fruit, and vegetables. Released by mast cells and basophils in the blood and tissues, after exposure to an allergen. Dilates blood vessels and makes them more permeable, to lower blood pressure.

Hormone. Biochemical sent as a messenger from one cell to another, often far away, traveling through the blood (*endocrine*) or into a duct and then into blood or directly into cell (*exocrine*). Many are produced in specialized glands, like the adrenals, pituitary, or thyroid, and in humans the signal to release them usually comes from the hypothalamus, a tissue located at the intersection of brain and spine and informed by sensors throughout the body.

Hyperactivity. Literally, too-high activity. Provoked by certain foods, stress, boredom, and so on, and possibly by pollutants, thyroid imbalance, or genetics. Part of *attention-deficit hyperactivity disorder (ADHD)*.

IgE. Immunoglobulin E. Antibody or receptor produced by certain immune cells in response to an allergen, then stored in plasma, other fluids, cell membranes, and so on. Its release triggers tissue cells to release inflammatory agents like histamine.

Immunotherapy. Rehabilitation of the immune system, often to resist a specific illness. Can be general, for example by bone marrow transplant, or specific, for example by gradually getting used to an allergen.

Intolerance. A physical and/or emotional, instant or delayed, local and/or systemic, mild or severe, non-life-threatening response to a food, substance, or non-substance. For example: diarrhea or headache from eating a certain food or poison, rash from touching a certain food or other substance, cough from breathing dust, and nausea from travel.

Kinesiology. Study of the anatomy and physiology of motion, and group of chiropractic methods, to detect and heal troubled nervous system responses to foods, other substances, and other stimuli. Also known as muscle testing.

Leukotriene. Type of inflammatory substance made from arachidonic acid, in white blood cells, and released during allergic reaction.

Mineral. Essential element, other than the carbon, hydrogen, nitrogen, and oxygen used to make most organic molecules, found in food and/or water. More or less of each dietary mineral, in balance with the others, is needed for the healthy functioning of cell and body processes. Those required in bulk are calcium, magnesium, phosphorus, potassium, sodium, and sulfur. Those needed in trace amounts include boron, cobalt, copper, fluorine, iodine, iron, manganese, molybdenum, selenium, zinc, and possibly chromium and some others.

Mutagenic. Regularly found to make cells produce inexact copies (mutations) when they replicate, or to accelerate an existing mutation. Caused by genetic damage.

Oral challenge. Trying a food that used to provoke allergy, to see if it still does.

Orthomolecular medicine. Therapy based on reducing excesses and supplementing deficiencies of vitamins, minerals, enzymes, amino acids, fatty acids, and other substances innate to our bodies.

Phenols. Group of aromatic chemical compounds suspected in intolerance or allergy. Most foods have some.

Placebo. Inert substance or treatment given as medicine to one group of people in a scientific study, to enable comparison with another group receiving an active substance or treatment.

Pollen. Powder of male sperm cells, in seed plants, able to be borne (typically, by wind or insects) to the female reproductive cells of plants of the same species.

Potentiation. Literally, empowerment. Increasing sensitivity to a fixed amount of an allergen, because of repeated exposure.

Prostaglandin. Group of substances, metabolized from fatty acids and vital to various body functions. Affect smooth muscle, inflammation, body temperature, and more. Type D-2 is an inflammatory agent derived from arachidonic acid.

Protein. Group of food and body substances made from amino acids. Vital to the structure and function of every cell in the body, and from there to build, metabolism, immunity, and reproduction. Animals and non-photosynthesizing plants must get it from food. Each kind of protein is a specific sequence of amino acids (*polypeptide chain*). The instructions for its assembly are genetically encoded.

Psychosomatic. Physical symptom created or intensified by emotion.

Salicylates. Subgroup of the phenol family of aromatic compounds, present in many fruit, vegetables, nuts, seeds, and other foods. Aspirin is a pure form of one of them.

Tachycardia. Racing heart.

Teratogenic. Regularly found to impair fetal development, leading to the appearance of birth defects.

Thromboxane. Type of inflammatory substance made from arachidonic acid, in blood platelets, and released during allergic reaction. Constricts blood vessels and promotes clotting.

Traditional Chinese medicine. System of foods, herbs, massage, acupuncture, and other tools to regulate body processes in relation to environmental influences. Organs and functions are grouped into five interacting elements (wood, fire, earth, metal, and water) and their energy is characterized in polarities like excessive-deficient, hot-cold, masculine-feminine, and interior-exterior.

Urticaria. Hives. Temporary condition of pale or reddened, itchy, raised patches of skin. Often caused by allergy.

Vaccination. Dose of a bacteria, virus, allergen, or other threat, in modified, weakened, or killed form, so that a person's immune system can still recognize it and know how to handle it, without being harmed by it, in the moment and, especially, upon future exposure. In other words, it stimulates the production of antibodies.

Vitamin. Group of substances found in foods and/or made in the body and needed in small amounts for various cell and body processes. Includes the fat-soluble vitamins A (*retinol*), D_1 (*ergocalcipherol*), D_2 (*calcipherol*), D_3 (*cholecalcipherol*), E (*alpha-tocopherol*), K_1 (*phylloquinone*), K_2 (*menaquinone*), K_3 (*menadione*), and

K$_4$ (*menadiol diacetate*), and the water-soluble vitamins B$_1$ (*thiamine*), B$_2$ (*riboflavin*), B$_3$ (*niacin*), B$_5$ (*pantothenic acid*), B$_6$ (*pyridoxine*), B$_7$ (*biotin*), B$_9$ (*folic acid*), B$_{12}$ (*cobalamin*), and C (*ascorbic acid*). The B and K vitamins need specific enzymes (*coenzymes*) to be present in order to function; A, C, D, and E do not.

The Sprouted Peanut Vaccine and Other Stories

Acknowledgments

If I am alive and well today, it is thanks in large part to my parents and brothers, Sandra, Richard, Jon, and Bruce, who have always looked out for me and from whose experiences I learn. Reading the words they wrote for you in Part Three, I am reminded how hard it has been for people like to them to protect people like me, and indeed to improve awareness and care of peanut allergy. Thanks too to my ancestors and relatives, including grandpas and grandmas Joe Gottlieb, Gina Obler, Jean Shizgal, and Jack Gollob.

Maya Goodrich, Holly MacKay, Jenni Huntly, and Justin Bur are friends who have been family in this and other ways. Françoise Giroux, David Dawson, Marilyn Gabriel, and Alain Morrier have been therapists and/or teachers of lasting value. Serge Rousseau was there for me in my most difficult years. Devlin Kuyek and Lucy Tomasetta keep being there for stimulating exchanges. Mélissa Guay humours my eyes, heart, and culture. Andrew Harwood and Nancy Stark Smith inspire growing by dancing. Alisha Piercy, Una & Fanon; Appiah Joseph Kojo Annan; Bruce Rutley; Coralie Malet; Delphine Marot; Eddie Fernandez Ureche, Biurys, Laura & Bryce; Francine Charpentier; Franc-Sois Dandurand; Hazel Letteen; Kavitro Roy; Lucy, Señora Rosa & Alfonso Arguello; Malcolm, Melanie, Sascha, and Oliver Clark; Orlando Rojas; Peter Wei Wang, Sunny, Cindy & Sophia; Rae Shepp; and William Archambault, Myriam Thomas, Florient & Simon, I am happy you too are here with me; Joel Ratcliffe, John Foster, Laurier Beauchamp, and Maira Martinez, I am also indebted.

This book began with small steps. Aurélie Brunelle, Chris Grollman, and Ivaylo Valtchev encouraged me to expand on earlier writings. Ken Dryden gave guidance on narrative nonfiction; Barry Burstein, access to periodical databases; and Carmen Lim, Catherine Crocker, Devlin, Ivaylo, and Lucy, feedback on drafts. Danielle Riome reminded me how much fun it can also be to have and read this kind of experience.

The Sprouted Peanut Vaccine and Other Stories

When I had what to publish but no experience with agents or publishers, Paula Kamen, author of *All in My Head: An Epic Quest to Cure an Unrelenting, Totally Unreasonable, and Only Slightly Enlightening Headache* (Da Capo Press), provided a model and introduction. Literary agent Beverley Slopen and Steven Forth of Indigo Books & Music also shared tips, and *Keep It Real: Everything You Need to Know about Researching and Writing Creative Nonfiction* (W. W. Norton), edited by Lee Gutkind, was a key resource.

In times of celebration as of discouragement, Bob Sinclair, Bruce Springsteen & the E Street Band, Daniela Mercury, Dumisani Maraire & Ephat Mujuru, the Flying Bulgur Klezmer Band, India Arie, Jack Johnson, Ry Cooder & Vishwa Mohan Bhatt, Wyclef Jean & Sak Pasé, *Maurice Richard, Talladega Nights,* and *The Lord of the Rings* grooved and soothed me, and showed how marvellously a person and team can develop.

As the rejection letters piled in, Devlin talked to me about self-publishing, and at first I wasn't too receptive. Then another book came along; being less controversial, about academic chemistry, it seemed fine to self-publish. Don Campbell and others at lulu.com taught me the ropes. Evan Perlman did a super job with the publicity and set things up for this endeavour.

By the time I came back to this project, it all had to be redone. Another, unexpected year. Meeting and then collaborating with illustrator Seán Newton was a turning point. I don't know how he reached inside and articulated what I saw, and am grateful for his devotion, presence, and fine teas. John Beasley Jr. of the University of Georgia Cooperative Extension Service helped us out with some peanut plant photos, Betsy Hageman of the National Association of Chain Drug Stores provided some info, Bill Nelson made some other photos, and Galen Bolland guided the presentation.

Only now do I understand how many other people have helped develop the awareness, writing, and body that go into this book:

Action Communiterre
Adam Pasamanick
Adrian Harewood
Aimée Darcel
Alex & Sarah Popivker
Ali & Café Rumi
Aliza Dwoskin
Allyna Harris
Amy Felske & family
Andrea del Moral
Andrew Bocarsly
Aniko Lysy
Anne Hoban
Asanti Dance Theatre
Association de contact-improvisation
Atef ben Hassen
Aux Vivres restaurant
Bahadur Bhatla
Basa family
Beatrice Lewis
Ben O'Hara-Byrne
Beto Hernandez
Bill Badger
Bob Bickford
Bruce Blake
Carl Barnes
Carl Freed
Carla Nemiroff
Carol Hayes
Geneviève Heistek
Geoff Selig
Gilles Crête
Gloria James
Harvey Michel
Helen Tudway-Cains
Hyacinth Young
Jackie Haas
James Pratt
Jane Browning
Janet Bourke
Jeannie Cronin
Jen Katz-Douek
Jin-Ran Kim
Joelle Bolduc
Johanna Mantsinen
John Campanelli
John Daly
Jon Wood
Judit Keri
Judy Wugalter
Julie Lebel
Juliet Huntly
KalmUnity
Kanehsatake Spiritual Gathering and Traditional Powwow
Ken Lum
Kern-Day family
Kevin Walsh
Kristen Dotti
La bottine aux herbes
Mary Thibault
Mauro Nobili & family
McGill Sports Camp
Michael Cooke
Michael Hayes
Michael Hurd
Michael Ross
Michelle Bowes
Miguel Veloza
Milton do Prado
Nadine Mondestin
Nancy Lawton
Nancy Paris
National Campus-Community Radio Association
Nick Foster
Oussou-Lio family
Paul Auster
Paul Pitchford
Pauline Brousseau
Pauline St-Mars
Peter Bunnell
Pey-Wen Ting
Phyllis Frederick
Pierre Loiselle
Pierre Minn
Rachel Kronick
Ranko Telebak
Rek Kwawer
Rob Gauvin
Robin Breger
Ron Feldman
Rose Enken

The Sprouted Peanut Vaccine and Other Stories

Carole Boucher
Carolyn Manzer
Carolyn Straub
Charles Lindsay
Chris Strachwitz
CKUT Radio McGill
Claire Lemieux
Clarence Johnson
Cornel West
Dahlia Genusov
Dave Berry
David Altmann
Debbie Mankovitz
Earthdance
Eden grocery
Elaine White
Élise Paquin
Ellen Gabriel
Emily Quant
Emmet Gowin
Ernesto Nobili & Spaccanapoli
Ferme Cadet-Roussel, Jean & Madeleine
François N'senga
Fredy Laverde
Frenco Vrac
Laura Karlin
Lena & Adam Atlas
Linda Morrison
Lisa Nelson
Loris Mirella
Louis Rigaud
Lourdes Pinedo
Lynda Raino
Mae Farinacci
Maitland Jones
Manon Paradis
Manu Kakkar
Marc Drouin
Margaret Enright
Marie, Denise, & Walter Sr. David & Susan Oke
Marie-Claude Gour, Pascal Larivière, Élodie & Félix
Marie-Hélène Grand'Maison
Marilyn Bronstein
Marjorie Carhart & Gyuri Hollosy
Mark Powell
Martha Stiegman
Mary & Herb Levitan
Rufo Valencia
Ryan Rutley
Sally Fallon
Samantha Burnell
Sandra Botnen
Sara Asher
Shannon Lynch
Sonia Osorio
Spirit Joseph
Steve Pitre
Studio 303
Sue Glover
Suzanne Plourde
Suzy Weber
Tade Fabumuyi Austine
Terrace Club
The Body Cartography Project
The Havurah
Thierno Diallo
Tim Lonn
Wayne Clasper
Winnie Larsen
Yves Léger
Yves Vial
Zyla Waters

Art and sport have been lifeblood and for this, even from a distance, you have changed and sustained me:

A. A. Milne
Ani Difranco
Berke Breathed
Bob Marley & the Wailers
Burning Sky
Carlos Vives
David Suzuki
Dead Can Dance
Dick Irvin Jr.
DJ Static & We Funk
Eduardo Galeano
Eurythmics
Fritjof Capra
G. S. Sachdev
Hockey Night in Canada

Howard Zinn
James Burke
John Hughes
Jorane
Kudsi Erguner
Mark Messier
Martin Cradick
Matt Groening & team
Mecca Normal
Mercedes Sosa
Michael Franti & Spearhead
Nos Canadiens de Montréal
P. G. Wodehouse

Primo Levi
Richard Desjardins
Sade
Sharon Burch
Socalled
Starhawk
Talib Kweli & DJ Hi-Tek
The '80s L. A. Lakers & '90s Chicago Bulls
Toni Morrison
U2
Warren Moon
Wayne Gretzky

Thanks even for what never clicked or went wrong; the confusion, fear, dislike, anger, humiliation, disappointment, and mourning that are as normal and valuable as the love, wonderment, hope, pleasure, victory, savouring, and rest.

The Sprouted Peanut Vaccine and Other Stories

Index

Acid-alkaline balance	71, 176, 192-193, 199
Adrenal glands	12, 27, 94, 97, 159, 191, 219
Adrenaline	3, 5, 9, 12, 36, 38, 59, 62, 107-108, 123, 140-141, 157-159, 172, 183, 191, 217
Aflatoxin	23, 36, 39-40, 44-45, 47, 50, 52, 64-65, 75, 78, 174, 176, 181, 184, 186, 189, 217
Agriculture	19-21, 23-24, 39-40, 44-45, 50-51, 67, 75. 79, 81, 95, 112, 115, 134, 137-138, 148-149, 151-152, 154, 161, 169, 175, 177, 179-180, 183-184, 191, 197, 199
Allergy	1, 3-6, 9-18, 20, 22-28, 33-85, 89-92, 98-103, 107-111, 113-116, 123, 130, 134-135, 139-152, 157-160, 163-166, 168-199
Anaphylaxis	1, 4, 9-12, 14, 35, 37-39, 41-43, 46, 58-59, 64-65, 74-78, 83-84, 107, 164, 169, 172-173, 179, 182, 187, 191, 217
Arachidonic acid	12, 22, 37-38, 45, 64, 79, 123, 176, 180, 217-218, 220-222
Aspirin – see Salicylates	
Asthma	1, 5, 11, 27, 39, 42, 45, 47, 49, 57-58, 61, 66, 70, 90, 100-101, 107-109, 123, 136, 164, 171, 173-174, 178, 182-183, 186, 188, 190, 199, 218
Attention Deficit Hyperactivity Disorder (ADHD) – see Hyperactivity	
Autism	5, 18, 49, 123, 141, 149, 218
Ayurveda – see Indian medicine	
Babies – see Early childhood	
Benadryl – see Diphenhydramine	
Blood type	67, 130-133, 191, 196
Body type – see Indian medicine	
Botany	19, 23-25, 40-41, 95, 180, 196, 198
Breastfeeding	26, 47, 50, 70, 84, 146, 186, 188-189
Cancer	5, 22-23, 32, 39-40, 52, 126, 134-138, 143-145, 147, 181, 184, 186, 196-199, 218-219, 221
Carbohydrate	17, 19, 21, 45, 57, 137, 145-147, 149, 165, 217-219

Children	3, 5-6, 9-11, 25, 31, 46-51, 57, 69-70, 85, 92, 95, 99, 101, 107, 116, 119-120, 141, 143, 153, 162, 169-173, 178-180, 183, 185-189, 195, 199

Chinese medicine – see Traditional Chinese medicine

Chronic fatigue	5, 123, 166
Cigarette smoke	39-40, 57, 64, 78, 80, 99-101, 118, 151, 181, 189, 217
Circulatory system	9, 38, 43, 45, 57, 64, 74, 94, 97, 111, 114, 123, 136, 143-144, 151, 163-164, 166, 172, 178, 191, 196, 199, 217, 219, 222
Cotton	21, 24, 35, 42-43, 67, 175, 177, 184
Dairy	5, 11, 23, 26, 35, 37-39, 44-45, 47, 49-52, 57, 70-71, 75, 115, 123, 131, 136, 138, 143, 146-147, 152, 177, 180, 182, 186, 188-189, 192, 197, 217, 219
Depression	5, 15, 17, 52, 89, 91, 95, 113, 123-124, 149, 164-166, 190, 219
Detoxification	24, 27, 61, 78, 80-81, 94, 135, 143, 190
Diphenhydramine	12, 54, 59-62, 141, 191, 218
Early childhood	10, 13, 25-27, 39, 46-47, 49-52, 57, 68-69, 75, 84-85, 95, 123-125, 139, 144, 146, 148, 153, 181, 186, 188-189, 195, 199, 222
Eczema	5, 11, 39, 42, 91, 124, 166, 171, 186, 218
Emotional reactions	1, 5, 10, 13, 28, 32, 46, 49, 52-53, 63, 70, 72, 74-76, 78, 84, 95, 98, 102, 120-121, 123, 141-143, 147, 151, 157-160, 164-165, 189-190, 222
Enzyme	11-12, 79, 89-90, 92, 135, 145, 149-150, 192, 196, 218, 221

Epinephrine – see Adrenaline

Evolution	6, 131, 140, 143-144, 147, 165, 178
Exercise	5, 17, 76, 79, 81, 83, 92, 109, 124, 135, 139, 160, 165-166, 177
Fat	19-22, 24-25, 27, 37-40, 44-45, 50-51, 57, 60, 63-65, 68, 71, 75, 79, 90, 132, 137-138, 143, 145, 149, 175-178, 180, 184, 192, 199, 219, 221-222
Favism	11, 103, 150, 198
Fish	5, 23, 35, 37, 41, 44-45, 51, 68, 75, 123, 131, 136-138, 180, 182, 197
Genetics	12, 19, 22, 24-25, 42, 44-45, 67, 119, 124-125, 130, 147, 174, 178, 183, 185, 198

Heart – see Circulatory system	
Herbal medicine	5, 10, 13, 61, 90, 95, 121, 166, 173, 186, 190
Histamine	5, 12, 14, 36, 39, 61, 89, 124, 135, 172, 191, 194, 218-220
History of peanut allergy	10-14
Hydrogenation	21, 45, 75, 178, 180
Hygiene hypothesis – see Sanitization	
Hyperactivity	5, 91, 123-124, 149, 164-165, 195, 220
Hypothalamus	12, 123, 159, 191, 217, 220
Immunoglobulin E (IgE)	11, 13-14, 36, 39, 41, 46, 49-52, 170, 185, 189-190, 193, 220
Immunotherapy	13, 38, 173
Indian medicine	24, 40, 66-67, 130-133, 177, 218
Infants – see Early childhood	
Intolerance	4, 10-11, 20, 39, 51-52, 57, 70, 74, 90, 100, 102, 143, 152, 170-171, 181, 188, 190, 195, 220
Kidneys	27, 43, 90, 94, 97, 145, 189, 196
Kinesiology	13, 90, 173, 220
Latex	5, 35
Leaky gut	28, 52, 71-72, 189
Legumes	5, 11-12, 19, 23-24, 34-40, 42, 44-45, 50-51, 55, 57, 63, 65-68, 80-81, 98-99, 103, 123, 131, 136-138, 142, 150, 152, 175-176, 180, 182-183, 186, 192-193, 197-198, 217
Leukotriene	12, 22, 38, 172, 220
Lifestyle	5, 12-13, 22, 26-28, 32, 42, 48-53, 57, 69-72, 76, 118, 130, 137, 145, 147, 165-166, 177
Liver	24, 27-28, 39, 43, 51-52, 61, 71, 80, 94, 99, 135-136, 143, 145, 150, 184, 189-190, 196
Medicine	3-5, 12-14, 20, 24, 28-29, 33, 35, 55, 57-59, 69, 77-78, 80, 83, 89-90, 94, 97, 115, 121, 123, 141, 150, 165, 168, 171-174, 189-190, 192, 199, 222
Milk – see Dairy	
Milk thistle	54, 59, 62, 143, 190
Minerals	19, 81, 90, 99, 102, 136, 145, 147, 150, 175, 192, 196, 220-221

Mold	5, 23, 27, 35, 39, 54, 56-57, 61, 63-64, 78, 98-101, 163, 176, 181, 193, 217
Muscle testing – see Kinesiology	
Noradrenaline	12, 172
Norepinephrine – see Noradrenaline	
Nutrition	5, 12-13, 21, 27, 42, 45, 49, 57, 64, 75, 81, 84, 90, 130, 134-138, 145-146, 152-153, 161, 165, 177, 179-181, 183, 186, 196-197
Nutritional supplements	81, 89-90, 161
Nuts	5, 9, 19, 23-24, 35-41, 45, 51, 55, 65-66, 68, 71, 122, 132, 136, 138, 170, 174-175, 180, 183, 185-186, 192, 217, 222
Orthomolecular medicine	89-90, 174, 194, 221
Peanut butter	21, 25, 45, 54, 65, 68, 71, 107, 169, 175-177, 180
Peanut oil	19-22, 37, 44, 63-64, 180, 184
Peanuts	1, 3-4, 6, 9-10, 13-17, 19-26, 29, 31-57, 59-60, 62-75, 77-79 81-85, 90, 92, 98, 101, 107-110, 113, 116, 118, 123, 134, 139-140, 142-143, 159, 164, 166, 168-186, 189-191, 193-194, 201-203, 217
Pesticides	24-25, 42-43, 67, 75, 177, 183-184, 192
Phenols	23, 38, 47, 64, 176, 181, 221-222
Phenylalanine	36, 123-124, 195
Pollen	5, 23-24, 35, 41-42, 45, 50, 66, 177, 182-183, 221
Pollution	5, 27, 49-50, 70, 75, 115, 171, 188-189
Potentiation	25, 39, 46, 68, 221
Pregnancy	13, 25, 46-47, 57, 68-69, 85, 114, 120, 186
Prostaglandin	12, 22, 38, 172, 221
Protein	11-13, 17, 19, 22, 36-38, 44-47, 49-50, 60, 63-64, 71, 75, 79, 84, 89-90, 119, 123, 137, 139, 143, 145, 147, 149-150, 166, 172, 174, 178-179, 184-186, 192-193, 197, 217, 219, 221-222
Psychosomatics – see Emotional reactions	
Radiation	26, 45, 48, 67, 69, 76, 174, 178, 185, 187
Roasting	20-21, 25, 36, 45, 56, 75, 137, 175, 177, 179
Salicylates	23, 35, 39, 64, 181, 222
Sanitization	27, 49, 51, 71, 75, 170, 178, 192

Scientific method	10, 30-33, 55
Seafood – see Shellfish	
Serotonin	124, 172, 195
Sex	5, 16, 57, 89, 94, 97, 99, 119, 123-126, 138, 143, 160, 165, 222
Shellfish	5, 35, 37, 45, 75, 123, 131, 137, 182, 217
Shiatsu	121, 142, 165, 169, 195
Sprouts	34, 45, 55-56, 63, 65, 68, 83, 92, 95, 98, 142, 177, 185, 193
Soy	12, 19, 35, 38, 40, 44-45, 50-51, 65, 80, 136-137, 175-176, 186, 192-193
Stings	11, 35, 41, 52, 157, 182
Tests for allergy	9, 14, 34, 54-57, 65, 83-85, 174, 183, 193
Thromboxane	12, 22, 38, 172, 222
Traditional Chinese medicine	4, 13, 28, 94, 97, 121, 138, 142, 165, 173-174, 192, 195, 222
Stress	5-6, 12, 15, 27, 49, 52, 71, 75, 80, 114, 123, 126, 142, 147, 161, 164-166, 193, 217-218, 220
Trauma	5, 15, 75, 112-113, 120, 141-142, 165
Vaccination	11, 13, 22, 26, 48-49, 51, 69, 75-76, 84, 187-188, 222
Vitamins	19, 44, 81, 89-90, 99, 135-136, 145, 178, 196, 221-223

Antibiotic exposure / Candida

Protein / arachidonic acid
overload IV/sp
79-80 - good suggestions
Supplements